# SAUNA SALVATION

## HARNESSING HEAT FOR PHYSICAL AND MENTAL HEALTH, SPIRITUAL REBIRTH, AND ENHANCED LONGEVITY

## DR. CYNTHIA MCCALLISTER

WORKSHOP OF
POSSIBILITY PRESS

# Medical Disclaimer

The information in "Sauna Salvation: Harnessing Intense Heat for Holistic Physical and Mental Health, Spiritual Rebirth, and Enhanced Longevity" is for educational and informational purposes only and is not intended to substitute for professional medical advice, diagnosis, or treatment. The practices discussed are scientifically informed and presented as examples of the potential benefits of heat exposure on physical and mental health and well-being. However, results can vary significantly between individuals.

Before incorporating suggestions from this book into your wellness practice, you are advised to consult with a healthcare professional. Intense heat has powerful effects on your body and should be approached cautiously, especially if you have a health condition or are pregnant. Get approval from your doctor before engaging in sauna practices to avoid potential health risks, especially if you have a pre-existing health condition, are pregnant, or are taking medications.

Always seek the advice of your physician or other qualified health provider with any questions you may have regarding a medical condition or before starting any new health regimen, including sauna use. Never disregard professional medical advice or delay seeking it because of something you have read in this book.

The author and publisher are not responsible for any adverse effects or consequences from using any suggestions, preparations, or procedures described in this book. The protocols featured in the book are suggested to individuals only, assuming medical approval has been obtained.

Reliance on any information this book provides is solely at your own risk. The author and publisher disclaim any liability based on this information for your decisions.

By reading this book and considering its contents, you acknowledge and agree that neither the author nor the publisher is liable for any injury, health impairment, or accident that may occur as a result of practicing sauna therapy or any other recommendations made herein.

This disclaimer applies to all content within "Sauna Salvation," including text, graphics, images, and other material.

First Edition

Published by Workshop of Possibility Press

1300 Post Road Ste 5

Fairfield, CT. 06824

ISBN: 978-1-941673-01-0 (Paperback)

ISBN: 978-1-941673-02-7 (Hardcover)

ISBN: 978-1-941673-03-4 (Ebook)

Library of Congress Cataloging-in-Publication Data

McCallister, Cynthia A.

p. cm.

Cover and interior design by Cynthia McCallister

Edited by Cynthia McCallister

Printed in the United States of America

2024

*This book is in remembrance of my beloved sister, Kathy, whose struggle to find peace compelled me to write it.*

———

*And with gratitude to my sauna sisters for connection and inspiration.*

# ACKNOWLEDGMENTS

With a heart full of gratitude, I extend my sincere thanks to the individuals and institutions that have made this work possible.

This book, born from the steam of countless sauna sessions over three years, owes its existence to the communities that welcomed me and provided space for my sauna practice at Sportsplex in Stamford, Connecticut, the Jewish Community Center in Woodbridge, and the Edge Fitness Club in Fairfield.

I am deeply grateful to my home institution, New York University's Steinhardt School of Culture, Education, and Human Development. The support, resources, and academic freedom it has afforded enabled this research, which connects scholarly inquiry with holistic wellness practices.

With deepest appreciation,
Cynthia McCallister

# About the Author

Dr. Cynthia McCallister is an Associate Professor of Teaching and Learning at the Steinhardt School of Culture, Education, and Human Development at New York University. Her research in applied behavioral science uniquely bridges educational theory with broader concepts of human well-being across the lifespan to emphasize continuous self-improvement.

**f** X 🄾

# 1. Introduction

In many cultures, particularly Scandinavia, sauna use is a deeply ingrained tradition. Many people engage in sauna sessions several times a week or even daily, typically spending 20 to 30 minutes in the heat to promote relaxation, well-being, and overall health.

In the depths of my struggle with a debilitating illness, I embarked on a personal journey that led me to discover the remarkable potential of the sauna as a tool for healing. In my journey, I employed the sauna daily for a much more prolonged time than is customary to reverse the devastating symptoms of my illness and to heal myself.

What began as a practice in self-care soon evolved into an extensive research project to explore the science of thermoregulation and the therapeutic potential of heat exposure so that I could develop a safe and effective protocol for extended-duration sauna practice.

This book reports the findings of my inquiry through a combination of insights from personal experience and scientific evidence. In it, I explain how extended heat exposure in the sauna mimics hot environmental conditions in which humans evolved and under which we function most optimally.

This book uncovers the fundamental processes of thermoregulation and explains how extended heat exposure potentially reverses disease processes, supports physical, mental, and spiritual well-being, and boosts longevity. Then, the book presents strategies and methods that you can weave into your own practice to increase your body's ability to withstand intense heat to improve wellness and longevity. I have tried and proven these methods through the evolution of my sauna practice.

**My Sauna Story**

Let me begin this book by sharing how I came to write it...

On the eve of my 60th birthday, I found myself in a state of severe chronic illness. My bodily systems and mental capacities had broken down at an alarming rate over the previous decade as a result of chronic stress and escalating mistreatment in an emotionally abusive and financially exploitative relationship of three decades. By that time, I was struggling with a constellation of ailments that included severe insomnia, chronic migraines, insulin resistance and obesity, extreme social anxiety, arrhythmia, bipolar depression, memory loss, and cognitive disorientation. I had been hospitalized for depression and suicidal ideations several years prior. Shortly after that, as my condition deteriorated, I had to take a four-month leave of absence from work due to my inability to execute complex tasks. I had become completely disabled. I was subsequently diagnosed with post-traumatic stress disorder (PTSD). Tests later confirmed I also suffered from adrenal gland dysfunction, severe dysbiosis (leaky gut), systemic inflammation, and metabolic imbalance.

Until then, I struggled blindly. Lacking insight into the root of the problem and being trapped in the toxic relationship, I attributed my declining health to genetics and aging. So, as symptoms developed, I sought medical attention, one specialist at a time, to provide a diagnosis and a prescription. By my 60th year, I was under the care of four physicians with multiple diagnoses, taking more than ten prescription medications. I couldn't function without pharmaceuticals, and to calm anxiety and sleep, I had become increasingly dependent on alcohol.

I don't exaggerate when I say that the sauna saved my life. After reading a scientific study that reported significant reductions in the risk of all-cause mortality through the use of the sauna, I decided to visit the dry sauna at my gym. I could tolerate the heat for only 10 minutes on my first visit. I visited again the next day and the day after, increasing the length of my sauna bath each day.

The effects were swift and remarkable. My mood lifted, sleep deepened, and I felt calmer and more at ease. However, the impact on my cardiovascular system astonished me the most. I'd recently taken up open-water swimming with seasoned endurance athletes in Long Island Sound. I'd committed to a grueling pool routine to keep pace: three vigorous hour-long interval sessions a week. Surprisingly, I found that sauna sessions matched the cardiac output of these intense swims without compromising my performance in the water. This discovery was a game-changer, offering a less taxing alternative to maintain my cardiovascular fitness.

Feeling better and becoming stronger, I continued ramping up heat exposure. Within a month, I was taking a daily 60-minute sauna bath in three 20-minute intervals alternating with minute-long cold showers. But my enthusiasm for getting more heat exposure was tempered with concern. As a newcomer to the sauna, I needed to familiarize myself with customary practices. Acquaintances at my gym who were more seasoned sauna bathers than I cautioned me against hour-long sessions, warning that such prolonged exposure is dangerous. Were they right?

**Sauna Inquiry**

Concerned about potential damage to my body through over-exposure to intense heat, I didn't break with sauna conventions recklessly. Instead, I transformed my sauna practice into an action research project with the hypothesis that extended-exposure sauna practice can prevent and reverse disease progression. I became a biohacker, testing my hypothesis through literature review and applying scientific principles to my practice. Through this research process, I developed a protocol for long-duration sauna practice.

Like most research, my sauna inquiry began with questions: How does the human body respond to heat? What are the benefits of heat exposure? How much heat can the body tolerate without causing damage?

My first pass through a few scientific studies on the effects of the sauna suggested that daily, 30-minute sessions dramatically reduce mortality risk and risk of cardiovascular disease. The studies were epidemiological, drawn from populations of sauna bathers in Scandinavia, where 30-minute sessions appeared to be custom. If 30-minute sessions reduce disease risk, longer 60-minute sessions might promise to reverse disease processes.

My professional life prepared me to take on this initiative. I'm a human development and learning scholar, a tenured professor at New York University, and an action researcher. In my work, I read and apply knowledge across philosophy and the behavioral and natural sciences to create innovative behavioral interventions that empower individuals to take the initiative to meet their goals and carry out their intentions (See McCallister, 2011 & 2022).

Driven by a thirst for scientific understanding, my expansive investigation touched down on the evolutionary origins of human thermoregulation, the cultural history of saunas, the intricate effects and therapeutic potential of heat stress on various bodily systems, and physiological responses to stress that enhance the strength and stillness of the psyche to promote mental wellbeing and consciousness. My experience ultimately led to understanding how sauna practice can be a sustaining spiritual practice.

Informed by continued research, I constantly adjusted my sauna protocol and increased my tolerance for exposure to heat. Today, more than three years after my first sauna visit, I practice a daily session of 90 minutes in a sauna of 180-190° Fahrenheit. My session is typically divided into three intervals of 50, 20, and 20 minutes, with periods of cooling off in the cold shower between intervals and after my session. During heat exposure intervals, I maintain a moderate-intensity heart rate lying on my back until the last five minutes, when I sit up and allow my heart rate to reach a higher zone. In experimenting with myself, I found that about 50 minutes of intense heat is needed before all of the sensations of tension dissipate and I am fully relaxed. Experiencing the relationship of

The aim of my sauna practice evolved through my experiment. My initial objective to identify the effects of heat on the bodily systems expanded to understand how heat exposure heightens the subjective sense of being. I'm a product of the Western approach to physical exercise to improve fitness and appearance. However, the psychic dimensions of my experience led me to appreciate ancient spiritual practices in which physical conditioning is pursued in the service of spiritual enlightenment. This research shows how heat exposure through sauna practice can be a powerful meditation and mindfulness practice.

My sauna experiment evolved beyond its initial scope, transforming from a study focused on heat's physiological effects into a broader exploration of its impact on consciousness and well-being. While I began with the typical Western perspective of physical conditioning for physical and aesthetic improvement, the profound psychic dimensions of my experience revealed unexpected parallels with ancient spiritual practices where improved physical fitness is a pathway to spiritual growth and self-discovery. My research demonstrates that sauna practice can be a potent tool for meditation and mindfulness, offering benefits that transcend physical conditioning.

### Self-transformation

Sauna practice has been a transformative turning point in my journey back to health. After three dedicated years of consistent practice, the cumulative effects are life-changing. One by one, most of the debilitating symptoms of bodily dysfunction disappeared. Once tormented by insomnia, I now sleep at least seven hours a night. After suffering from tachycardia for more than a decade, my resting heart rate is now 67 beats per minute. I'm no longer insulin-resistant, and my weight is normal. My key vitals, such as my A1C and cholesterol profile, are normal. Persistent migraines have ceased. My immunity improved; I haven't had a cold or infection in several years. I've come off most prescription medications.

Beyond physical rejuvenation, sauna practice has restored my mental and emotional well-being. Addictive impulses have faded, allowing me to exist in the present with a new sense of contentment. As persistent anxiety quieted, my mood stabilized, and I could experience life from a more stable place of calm and self-assurance. A renewed focus and mental clarity enhance my ability to carry out my intentions in my personal and professional life.

### Navigating this Book

This book invites you to embark on a journey of self-discovery and transformation through sauna practice tailored to your unique needs.

To that end, I encourage you to read the book in a way that is relevant to your journey. The first four chapters are universally applicable, providing a basic understanding of human thermoregulation and the rich history behind sauna practice. The chapters in Section II are specific to bodily functions and the therapeutic potential of heat in improving dysregulation. You can selectively read relevant chapters depending on your wellness goals or the health challenges you face.

You'll notice repetition throughout Section III. This is intentional because the cellular-level physiological processes of the body's heat response described in the section's first chapter play a part in the therapeutic effects of heat on various body systems discussed in each subsequent chapter.

When you are ready to begin your practice, the chapters in Section III explain how to establish a routine for using the dry sauna for cardiovascular endurance training to reap the benefits of cellular cleansing and revitalization. While the principles and benefits of heat therapy apply to other sources, such as steam rooms and infrared saunas, dry saunas are the best option for our purposes. Compared to infrared saunas, the heart rate can be raised more effectively in dry saunas due to their higher temperatures, which cause greater cardiovascular stress and a more intense body cooling response. While steam rooms are hot enough to raise heart rate significantly, they are less suited for prolonged workouts due to their high humidity and the body's inability to cool through evaporative sweating.

Once sauna practice has become part of your routine, you will begin to notice and reap the benefits of heat to mental well-being. The chapters in Section IV guide you in aiming your practice objectives toward achieving inner peace and spiritual awakening.

**Productive Skepticism**

While transformative in my experience, sauna therapy may evoke skepticism in some—a healthy attitude in today's landscape of quick fixes and miracle cures. While the sauna was a catalyst for my holistic improvement, I encourage critical thinking and respect for scientific evidence when considering any health practice.

While it's essential to approach any wellness practice with a discerning eye, the evidence suggests that sauna therapy can be a powerful tool for holistic well-being. By balancing traditional wisdom with current, peer-reviewed research, this book offers a comprehensive, evidence-based exploration of sauna therapy that empowers readers to make informed decisions about its role in their wellness routines.

**Conclusion**

As you begin to implement the practices outlined in this book, you may find yourself experiencing a range of benefits: improved health, increased energy, better sleep, heightened self-awareness, greater resilience in the face of life's challenges, and a stronger connection to your body's innate wisdom. Regardless of your age, physical condition, or any health issues you may be facing, sauna practice can become a transformative element in your life—perhaps one of the most meaningful gifts you've given yourself.

# PART ONE

## THE HUMAN RELATIONSHIP TO HEAT

Human beings have an intricate and profound connection with heat shaped by millions of years of evolution and thousands of years of cultural development. Heat has played a crucial role in our survival and development as a species.

The chapters in this section will provide a foundation for understanding the numerous health benefits of sauna practice. Chapter Two explores how humans acquired exquisitely developed thermoregulatory capacities through evolution.

Heat has played a significant role in human cultures around the globe. Chapter Three explores how diverse cultures have developed practices to use heat for therapeutic, spiritual, and social purposes.

Chapter Four delves into the human physiological response to heat and explores its effects on various body systems. This knowledge is foundational for understanding the therapeutic effects of sauna practice on each body system, which are the topics of chapters in Section III.

Understanding the adaptive, cultural, and physiological significance of the human relationship to heat will help you establish a firm foundation for developing your sauna practice.

# 1. Heat and Human Evolution

E volution, driven by natural selection, shapes species to fit their ecological niches over time. Organisms with beneficial traits for their environment survive and reproduce more successfully.

Nature gave humans remarkable adaptability to temperature extremes to survive and thrive in extreme temperatures. This chapter explores our distinctive physical traits and behavioral adaptations for thermoregulation. Knowledge of our heat adaptability will help explain how prolonged exposure to intense heat causes the body to respond in ways that stimulate thermoregulation processes, enabling it to strengthen and protect itself. So, let's begin an investigation into how our extraordinary thermoregulatory capacities came into being.

### *In the beginning...*

Humans began developing as a species as herbivores who hunted and gathered in cooperative partnerships. They initially consumed a varied diet, including insects, scavenged foods from predator kills, and plants. But over time, as they adapted to different environments and developed skills and tools for hunting, their diet shifted to include more animal products, eventually reaching a *hypercarnivorous* level on the food chain, meaning that more than 70% of their diet consisted of animal sources (Ben-Dor, Sirtoli & Barkai, 2021).

Until approximately 80,000 years ago, before the extinction of numerous large animal species, humans held the role of apex hunters positioned at the pinnacle of the food chain. They achieved this through mastery of persistence hunting, a method involving chasing prey until it tires and succumbs to exhaustion.

Humans acquired several distinctive traits for persistent hunting, such as social-cognitive capacities to participate in large social groups to pool the knowledge and expertise required to coordinate hunting.

Persistence hunting requires chasing prey over long distances. Humans developed the capacity for endurance running some two million years ago (Bramble & Lieberman, 2004). Some estimates suggest they could run 20 to 40 kilometers (12 to 25 miles) per day during hunts and, in extreme cases, might have pursued prey over two or more days, potentially covering up to 80 kilometers (50 miles).

### Thermoregulation: An Evolutionary Triumph

Persistence hunting requires running during the strongest heat of the day when other predators are less active. Humans spent a significant part of their evolutionary history in East Africa, including modern-day Kenya, where, according to Passey et al. (2010), temperatures have been consistently high, with an average of around 95°F over the past 4 million years. This stable, hot environment may have influenced human adaptation and improved capacity to regulate body temperature and safely tolerate extreme heat.

Understanding these traits helps us understand why, with proper conditioning, the body can safely endure high temperatures like those in the dry sauna.

### Body Shape and Size

The shape and size of the human body evolved for better heat dissipation. Compared to other primates, humans are relatively tall with longer limbs, which increases the surface area relative to body volume. This higher surface area-to-volume ratio helps with more efficient heat loss.

### Bipedalism

Bipedalism, or the ability to walk on two legs, allows for more efficient cooling by minimizing solar heat absorption and maximizing heat dissipation. With less body mass exposed directly to the sun and the head and torso positioned higher above the earth's surface, a smaller surface directly faces the sun's rays. Bipedalism also reduces metabolic heat production, or the amount of heat expended during locomotion, compared to quadrupedal knuckle-walking.

### Human Skin and Sweating Capacity

As early humans migrated into Africa's hot, open savannas, their skin underwent significant changes to better cope with the increased exposure to heat and sunlight. Unlike most other animals, human skin is naked. While lack of fur exposes us to the elements, less hair allows for more effective sweating. With less insulation, moisture can evaporate more freely from the skin, allowing for more direct heat loss from the skin to the environment.

Another notable adaptation was the development of a more efficient sweating system. The skin's sweat glands in the dermis became more numerous and active. When exposed to heat, these glands secrete sweat onto the skin's surface, which evaporates, cooling the body and preventing overheating.

The skin's structure also evolved to enhance heat dissipation. The *dermal papillae*, tiny finger-like projections of the dermis, the inner layer of skin, into the epidermis, the outer layer, became more pronounced, increasing the surface area for heat exchange between the skin and the environment.

Developing a more complex melanin production system is another significant adaptation in the skin. Melanin, the pigment that causes skin color, is produced by melanocytes in the epidermis. As early humans spent more time in open, sun-exposed environments, their skin adapted to produce more melanin, providing better protection against the harmful effects of ultraviolet radiation. This adaptation helped to reduce the risk of skin damage and ensure the survival and reproductive success of individuals with more protective skin pigmentation.

The increased heat exposure also likely influenced the development of a more efficient cardiovascular system. The dermis contains a network of blood vessels that play a vital role in thermoregulation. When the body needs to cool down, these vessels dilate, increasing blood flow to the skin and releasing more heat into the environment.

### Deliberate Hydration

Because humans have the capacity for conscious awareness, they can be cognizant of thirst. Mindful awareness of thirst and deliberate water consumption allowed humans to regulate and maintain water balance in hot environments.

### Cultural Ingenuity and Behavioral Thermoregulation

Lastly, humans have developed behavioral and cultural practices to regulate temperature. For example, using fire to cook foods has reduced the need for internal metabolic heat production. Also, the development of heating technologies has enabled humans to create high-intensity heat environments, like saunas, for comfort, healing, and spiritual practice.

### Conclusion

Evolutionary adaptations have granted us the gift of coping effectively with excess heat. The sauna is a special space that reconnects us with the origins of our remarkable human thermoregulatory capacities by providing a controlled environment that exposes the skin to high temperatures, activating physiological mechanisms that developed to allow our species to thrive in diverse environmental conditions.

Although sauna bathing at temperatures ranging from 80-100°C (176-212°F) certainly pushes the body beyond its usual thermal comfort zone, our sophisticated thermoregulatory system is capable of maintaining a stable core temperature and preventing hyperthermia, even during extended sauna sessions.

As you embark on your sauna journey, know that consistent practice can awaken dormant thermoregulatory superpowers deep within your DNA. With continued exposure to heat, your body will adapt and grow stronger, gradually unlocking your innate ability for thermal thriving.

# 2. Heat Stress and Thermoregulation: Physiological Mechanisms and Responses

T he human body's ability to maintain a stable internal temperature in the face of varying environmental conditions is a testament to the intricate interplay of its organ systems. This thermoregulatory capacity showcases the remarkable coordination between different biological levels of organization, from cells to organs to entire systems.

This chapter will explore how various body systems contribute to temperature regulation. By examining each system's role in thermoregulation, we'll understand how the body maintains homeostasis in response to temperature challenges. This exploration will highlight the interconnectedness of our physiological processes and their collective effect on preserving overall health.

### Thermoregulatory Responses at the Cellular Level

Sauna therapy induces controlled heat stress that triggers beneficial adaptations deep within the body's cells. Heat stress from the sauna can stimulate the expression of heat shock proteins (HSPs), which play a crucial role in keeping proteins in the cells in good repair. Proteins are the cell's workhorses, carrying out all its functions. HSPs also contribute to systemic thermoregulation by protecting vital organs and tissues from heat damage.

The mild oxidative stress caused by the sauna's heat can strengthen the body's antioxidant defenses, enhancing the body's natural capacity to neutralize free radicals and manage oxidative stress more effectively. Free radicals are unstable molecules that can damage cells. Sauna-induced heat stress also positively influences mitochondrial function.

Mitochondria, the specialized structures within cells responsible for producing energy in the form of ATP (adenosine triphosphate) through a process called cellular respiration, are significantly influenced by sauna therapy. The heat stress from sauna use can improve mitochondrial efficiency, stimulate mitochondrial biogenesis, and enhance ATP production.

Additionally, regular sauna use stimulates autophagy, a cellular "housekeeping" process that removes damaged components and enhances stress resistance.

These cellular adaptations work together to improve overall resilience, potentially contributing to better cardiovascular function, enhanced detoxification, boosted immune function, and positive effects on mental health. The controlled heat stress from sauna use thus initiates a series of beneficial adaptations at the cellular level, highlighting its potential as a tool for health maintenance and performance optimization.

**Thermoregulatory Response of the Nervous System**

The nervous system is crucial in regulating body temperature during sauna use. The central component of the thermoregulatory system is the hypothalamus, a small region located between the top of the brain stem and beneath the thalamus. The hypothalamus is the primary control center, receiving and processing information about the body's temperature and initiating appropriate responses to maintain homeostasis.

Thermoreceptors are specialized sensory receptors distributed throughout the skin, organs, and blood vessels that continuously monitor the body's thermal environment and sense changes in temperature. In the heat of the sauna, thermoreceptors send signals to the hypothalamus.

Upon receiving these signals, the hypothalamus activates the autonomic nervous system, which consists of the sympathetic and parasympathetic divisions. The sympathetic nervous system is primarily responsible for the body's thermoregulatory responses in the sauna. It stimulates the dilation of blood vessels in the skin, a process known as vasodilation, which increases blood flow to the skin's surface and facilitates heat dissipation from the body to the environment, helping to prevent overheating.

The sympathetic nervous system also activates the sweat glands, increasing perspiration and evaporation of sweat from the skin's surface to remove heat and lower body temperature. The autonomic nervous system also modulates metabolic processes, such as increasing heart and respiratory rates, to support the body's increased demand for oxygen and nutrients during heat stress.

The parasympathetic division of the autonomic nervous system helps to counterbalance the effects of the sympathetic nervous system. It promotes vasodilation in certain blood vessels, such as those in the gastrointestinal tract, to redirect blood flow to the skin for cooling. The parasympathetic nervous system also regulates sweat gland activity and helps conserve energy and maintain normal bodily functions during sauna use.

The hypothalamus continuously monitors the body's temperature through feedback from thermoreceptors and makes necessary body-wide adjustments to maintain thermal equilibrium.

**Thermoregulatory Response of the Integumentary (Skin) System**

*Integument* means the tough outer layer. The body's outer protective layer of skin, the integumentary system, is the largest organ in the body. It accounts for 15% of total body weight, with an average surface area in adults of about 1.7 square meters, or just under 18 square feet. The skin helps to protect against disease, dehydration, and over-exposure to the sun. It's the body's system for sensing and feeling its way in the environment. We experience tactile sensations through the skin, transmitted via the nervous system, guiding our movements and interactions within the world around us.

In addition to serving as a sensory interface to the environment and providing protection from it, the skin is also a powerful heat regulator and cooling system, providing a large area for heat exchange between the body and the environment. In the sauna, where ambient temperatures can reach 100°C (158-212°F), exposure to intense heat causes the skin temperature to rise rapidly. Thermoreceptors in the skin signal the hypothalamus, which responds to these signals by initiating cooling mechanisms of thermoregulation and the release of excess heat to prevent overheating. These processes involve the production of sweat and the dilation or constriction of blood vessels.

### Sweat and evaporative cooling

The skin is laden with eccrine sweat glands of two main types: eccrine glands and apocrine glands. Eccrine glands, found all over the body, produce most sweat. Eccrine glands consist of a secretory coil and a duct that opens onto the skin's surface through a pore. When exposure to the extreme heat of the sauna causes the body's temperature to rise, the hypothalamus stimulates the sweat glands to produce sweat.

Sweat is mostly water with small amounts of electrolytes such as sodium, potassium, and chloride. Sweating is one of the primary ways the body cools itself. As the sweat evaporates from the skin, it takes heat away from the body. This process is known as *evaporative cooling*. Through sweating and evaporation, heat dissipates effectively, allowing for prolonged physical activity in the searing heat. This evaporative cooling is crucial in maintaining the body's core temperature within a safe range during protracted exposure to high heat.

Humans have a much higher density of sweat glands in their skin compared to other animals. For example, humans possess over ten times the number of sweat glands per area unit of skin than chimpanzees, our closest living relatives.

### Vascular control

The skin is highly vascularized, with a network of blood vessels that can dilate or constrict to regulate blood flow and heat exchange. In response to heat stress, blood vessels, especially those near the skin, called capillaries, widen in a process known as vasodilation, described in the section below. This increase in blood vessel diameter allows more blood to flow to the skin, where heat can be released into the environment, helping to cool the body down.

Humans can both increase or decrease blood flow to the skin. In cold environments, vasoconstriction reduces blood flow to the skin, conserving body heat. This ability to adjust blood flow helps maintain core body temperature within a narrow, optimal range in various environmental conditions.

**Thermoregulatory Response of the Cardiovascular System**

The cardiovascular system, which includes the heart and blood vessels, is essential for regulating body temperature during sauna use. Its primary role is distributing oxygen, heat, and nutrients throughout the body.

The cardiovascular system is highly adaptable, allowing the body to adjust to different conditions, such as heat and increased physical activity, through *vasodilation* (widening of blood vessels) and *vasoconstriction* (narrowing of blood vessels).

The key to this adaptability lies in the adjustments made to cardiac output, which is the amount of blood pumped by the heart per minute. Two factors determine cardiac output: *heart rate* (the number of times the heart beats per minute) and *stroke volume* (the volume of blood pumped out with each heartbeat). When either or both of these factors increase, cardiac output also increases. This increase in cardiac output is vital in situations like heat exposure or physical activity, where the body needs more oxygen and nutrients to function properly.

During sauna use, the hypothalamus signals the heart to increase its rate, a response known as *tachycardia*. An increased heart rate allows more blood to be pumped throughout the body, enhancing heat transport from the core to the skin's surface for dissipation.

The cardiovascular system also adjusts *blood pressure* to support thermoregulation. In the sauna, dilating blood vessels in the skin can temporarily drop blood pressure. This process occurs because the dilated vessels have a larger diameter, accommodating a greater blood volume. Consequently, the pressure within the vessels may temporarily drop since the same amount of blood is distributed over a larger space.

The cardiovascular system compensates to counteract the potential drop in blood pressure and ensure adequate blood flow to vital organs. The heart, in particular, increases its *contractile force*. Contractile force is the force generated by the contraction of the heart muscle fibers. By increasing the force of contraction, the heart can pump blood more effectively, helping to maintain blood pressure within a normal range.

Cold exposure after sauna use can lead to a temporary increase in blood pressure due to the body's physiological response to the sudden change in temperature. When exposed to cold, the blood vessels near the skin's surface constrict (vasoconstriction) to minimize heat loss and preserve core body temperature. This constriction increases peripheral resistance, forcing the heart to work harder to pump blood through the narrowed vessels, resulting in a temporary rise in blood pressure. Additionally, cold exposure triggers the activation of the sympathetic nervous system, which releases hormones like adrenaline and noradrenaline, further contributing to the increase in heart rate and blood pressure.

**Thermoregulatory Response of the Muscular System**

While the sauna environment primarily challenges the body's ability to dissipate heat, the thermoregulatory system also employs mechanisms to generate heat when necessary. These heat generation processes, including shivering and non-shivering thermogenesis, are typically associated with cold exposure but can also play a role in maintaining thermal balance during sauna use, particularly during the cooling-down phase or in the event of a sudden temperature drop.

Shivering is a heat-generation mechanism that involves the rapid contraction of skeletal muscles. In exposure to cold temperatures, peripheral thermoreceptors throughout the body signal the hypothalamus to initiate the shivering response. During shivering, skeletal muscles throughout the body contract and relax in a rapid, rhythmic manner. These contractions require energy released in the form of heat. The generated heat helps to warm the body and maintain core temperature. Shivering can be an effective short-term response to cold exposure. Still, it isn't a sustainable long-term solution, as it can be energy-intensive and may interfere with other bodily functions.

In addition to shivering, the body generates heat through non-shivering thermogenesis, primarily in brown adipose tissue (BAT), also known as brown fat. BAT is a specialized type of fat rich in mitochondria, the cellular organelles responsible for energy production. Unlike white adipose tissue, which stores energy, BAT's primary function is to generate heat. In response to cold exposure, the sympathetic nervous system releases norepinephrine, a neurotransmitter that binds to receptors on BAT cells. This binding triggers a series of metabolic processes that result in the breakdown of stored fat and heat generation. The heat generated by BAT helps to warm the blood circulating through it, which then distributes the heat throughout the body.

Non-shivering thermogenesis in BAT may not be a primary heat generation mechanism during sauna use when the body works to dissipate heat. However, BAT activation occurs in exposure to cool environments, such as during the cooling-down phase between sauna intervals and at the end of a session.

Incorporating cold exposure into your sauna practice with a cold shower or cold plunge collectively stimulates mitochondrial biogenesis, activates uncoupling proteins, enhances substrate oxidation, and triggers *hormetic* effects—the beneficial physiological responses triggered by exposure to low doses of stressors. These effects increase energy production and efficiency in mitochondria.

**Thermoregulatory Response of the Respiratory System**

The respiratory system, which includes the nasal passages, throat, and lungs, is primarily responsible for gas exchange and oxygenation of the body. However, the respiratory system can contribute to heat loss through evaporative heat loss, when moisture in the lungs and airways evaporates during breathing, absorbing heat from the body and helping to cool it as the water vapor is exhaled. This process is triggered when the hypothalamus in the brain signals the respiratory system to increase the breathing rate. An elevated breathing rate, known as *tachypnea*, allows for more rapid air exchange between the lungs and the environment.

As air passes through the nasal passages and throat, it comes into contact with the moist mucous membranes lining these structures. The high ambient temperature in the sauna causes the moisture on these surfaces to evaporate, absorbing heat from the surrounding tissues. This evaporative cooling effect helps to lower the temperature of the blood circulating through the respiratory tract, which then distributes the cooled blood throughout the body.

In addition to the nasal passages and throat, the lungs contribute to respiratory evaporative heat loss. The lungs contain a large surface area of moist, highly vascularized tissue, making them efficient sites for heat exchange. As air moves in and out of the lungs during breathing, it picks up moisture from the lung surfaces. The evaporation of this moisture absorbs heat, helping to cool the blood circulating through the lungs.

The rate and depth of breathing can influence the amount of heat lost through the respiratory tract. Individuals may naturally adopt a slightly faster and deeper breathing pattern during sauna to enhance heat loss. This increased ventilation allows a greater air volume to pass over the respiratory surfaces, facilitating more efficient evaporative cooling.

The respiratory system plays a more significant role in thermoregulation in some animals, such as dogs. These animals often engage in panting, a rapid, shallow breathing pattern that maximizes airflow over the moist surfaces of the tongue, mouth, and respiratory tract. Panting allows for a high evaporation rate and efficient heat loss, helping these animals cool down in hot environments. However, panting isn't a primary thermoregulatory mechanism in humans and is less efficient than sweating for heat dissipation.

### Thermoregulatory Response of the Endocrine System

The endocrine system, a network of glands that produce and secrete hormones, regulates various physiological processes, including thermoregulation. Hormones, the chemical messengers of the endocrine system, work in concert with the nervous system to influence metabolic rate, heat production, and the body's response to stress. Several key hormones and endocrine axes contribute to maintaining thermal balance in sauna use.

Thyroid hormones, produced by the thyroid gland, are essential regulators of metabolic rate and heat production. During sauna use, the increased metabolic activity induced by thyroid hormones can contribute to the body's overall heat production, helping to maintain core temperature in the face of heat stress.

The adrenal glands atop the kidneys also play a significant role in thermoregulation by producing epinephrine (adrenaline) and norepinephrine (noradrenaline) in response to stress. Epinephrine and norepinephrine activate the sympathetic nervous system, triggering a range of physiological responses that support thermoregulation. Epinephrine and norepinephrine stimulate the dilation of blood vessels in the skin, enhancing blood flow and facilitating heat dissipation. They also increase heart rate and contractility, ensuring adequate circulation and delivery of oxygen and nutrients to the body's tissues. Furthermore, these hormones stimulate sweat gland activity, promoting perspiration and evaporative cooling. The combined effects of epinephrine and norepinephrine help the body regulate its temperature during sauna use.

The hypothalamus-pituitary-adrenal (HPA) axis, a complex endocrine pathway, also plays a role in thermoregulation and the body's response to stress. The hypothalamus, the central regulator of the HPA axis, integrates information about the body's thermal state and initiates appropriate hormonal responses. When exposed to heat stress, such as in the sauna, the hypothalamus stimulates the pituitary gland to release adrenocorticotropic hormone (ACTH).

ACTH, in turn, stimulates the adrenal glands to produce and secrete cortisol, a glucocorticoid hormone with wide-ranging effects on metabolism, immune function, and stress adaptation. Cortisol helps mobilize energy reserves, such as glucose, to support the body's increased metabolic demands during heat stress. It also has anti-inflammatory properties, helping to protect tissues from potential damage induced by the sauna's high temperatures.

**Conclusion**

The human body's ability to maintain a stable internal temperature is a marvel of biological engineering. Through an intricate network of sensors, feedback loops, and effector mechanisms, our thermoregulatory system allows us to function effectively across a wide range of environmental conditions.

# 3. The History and Tradition of the Sauna

As humans ventured into the world's colder regions, they developed technologies to trap intense heat for physical exposure at adequate levels to stimulate the physiological processes explained in the last chapter. These technologies were humanity's first saunas.

Archeologists have discovered structures similar to what we now know as the sauna—dwellings in which rocks are heated to produce intense heat—that date back thousands of years. The earliest evidence of saunas dates back to around 7000 BCE in Northern Europe, in the areas that are now Finland and the Baltic countries. These early saunas were simple pits dug into slopes in the ground, with a fireplace where stones were heated to high temperatures. Water was thrown on the hot stones to produce steam and create a hot, humid environment. Saunas were used for cleansing, relaxation, and ritual purposes.

Iron Age saunas dating back to the fourth century BCE were discovered in excavations in Stone Age hill forts of the Northwest Iberian Peninsula. Archeologists have also found evidence of a community sauna in the excavations of an ancient Mayan village that is 1,400 years old. The oldest Roman baths in Asia Minor were discovered in Sagalassos, Turkey, dating back to 10 AD.

As civilizations developed, saunas spread across continents. In Scandinavia, saunas became commonplace among the Vikings, who incorporated them into daily routines and took them on their voyages, seeding heat therapy technology into cultures worldwide. The first written mention of saunas appears in Arab texts, describing the bathing habits of Vikings and Slavic peoples.

The rest of this chapter delves into the rich traditions of heat utilization across global cultures to show how humans have ingeniously harnessed heat for health and healing.

### Finnish Sauna

A Finnish sauna is a small, wooden room designed for dry or wet heat sessions. It's typically constructed of a wooden interior with walls, ceilings, and benches made of softwoods like pine, spruce, or aspen. The wood creates a soothing, aromatic atmosphere.

Traditionally heated with wood, most modern saunas are heated with electric or gas-powered furnaces, often with rocks piled on top. Water is thrown on the rocks to create steam and control humidity. hat water is poured on to raise the temperature to the desired level. Temperatures can reach up to 70–100°C (158–212°F). There are typically two or three benches for sitting or lying down. The higher benches are hotter as heat rises.

Lighting in the sauna is usually dim to create a relaxing ambiance. Sauna accessories include buckets or ladles and thermometers. Birch whisks ("vihta" or "vasta") are sometimes used to gently beat the body, which improves circulation and exfoliates the skin. The door is typically made of wood and has a small window or gap at the bottom to regulate airflow. The sauna room is usually connected to a dressing room or shower area where people can cool off after their sauna session.

### Russian Banya

A *banya* is a traditional Russian steam bath, similar to a sauna, but with some distinct characteristics. It typically consists of a small wooden building or room designed for wet or dry heat sessions, followed by a cool rinse or plunge into cold water. Like the Finnish sauna, banyas are usually heated by a wood-burning stove with rocks placed on top. Water is poured on the rocks to generate steam. The *venik*, a bundle of dried birch, oak, or eucalyptus twigs, is used to gently beat the body, which improves circulation and exfoliates the skin. After the heat session, people often cool down by taking a plunge into cold water or snow or simply by stepping outside. The banya is a significant part of Russian culture and social life, and it is often enjoyed with friends and family.

## Roman Baths

The history of the Roman bath played a central role in ancient society, culture, and daily life. The Romans recognized heat baths' therapeutic and social benefits and constructed elaborate public bathhouses throughout their empire. The Roman baths were large complexes open to the community where people gathered to bathe in heated and cooled rooms and to socialize, exercise, and bathe in water. The Roman baths included a warm room (Caldarium), a hot room, similar to what we now know to be a sauna (Laconicum), and a natatorium, or a room with a cold bath (Frigidarium).

These baths were massive in scale, capable of accommodating hundreds of bathers simultaneously. In addition to bathing facilities, they featured libraries, gymnasiums, and gardens. The architecture of the baths reflected Roman engineering prowess, with vast vaulted ceilings, intricate mosaics, and sophisticated heating systems known as *hypocausts*.

The Roman tradition of public baths, centered around heating and cooling the body, eventually disappeared in the West with a transition to public bathing facilities emphasizing physical hygiene.

## Turkish Baths

In the Middle East, North Africa, Central Asia, and the Indian subcontinent, the Roman baths were adapted to meet the needs of the Islamic world, where the *hammam*, or Turkish bath, provided not only a place to seek heat, cleanse, and socialize but to carry out the ritual cleansing before prayer in the Islamic religion. The hammam experience involves moving into increasingly warmer rooms, typically heated by steam, exfoliation with a special glove called a *kese*, a massage with aromatic oils, and finishing by washing under warm water. There is no cold exposure.

Over the centuries, hammams became integral to Ottoman social life and architecture. As the Ottoman Empire expanded across Southeast Europe, the Middle East, and North Africa, the hammam became a staple of urban life in many conquered cities, becoming integrated into the daily routines of diverse populations.

These baths were meticulously designed with stunning architecture, featuring domed ceilings, intricate tilework, and marble interiors. The layout typically included separate sections for men and women, each equipped with hot and cold rooms and massage and relaxation areas.

In contemporary times, the rise of wellness culture has further cemented Turkish baths' place in global cities as sites for relaxation, beauty treatments, and social gatherings. Today, Turkish baths are found in major cities around the world.

### Native American Sweat Lodge

The history of Native American sweat lodges traces back thousands of years and is deeply rooted in indigenous cultures across North America. Traditionally, the sweat lodge is constructed with a framework of saplings covered by hides, blankets, or other materials, creating a low-domed enclosure. Rocks, often heated in a fire outside the lodge, are brought inside and placed in a central pit. Water is then poured over these hot stones, producing steam and raising the temperature inside the lodge. Participants sit in a circle around the stones, engaging in prayers, chants, or other rituals as they undergo the intense heat and sweat.

Throughout history, the sweat lodge has served as a place of physical, mental, and emotional cleansing for Native American peoples, and the sweat lodge ceremony is considered a central aspect of spiritual and communal life. It is believed to facilitate a deep connection with the natural world, the spirit realm, and the inner self. The experience of sweating and purging is seen as a symbolic and spiritual purification, helping individuals to release negative energy, trauma, and illness.

### Japanese Onsen

An *onsen* is a Japanese hot spring around which bathing facilities and inns are often situated. As a volcanically active country, Japan has thousands of onsens scattered throughout its major islands. Traditionally, onsens were public bathing places. They are publicly run by a municipality or privately run, often as part of a hotel or bed and breakfast. Onsens come in many types and shapes, including outdoor and indoor baths. The water in an onsen can have a variety of mineral compositions, which provide different health benefits.

### Korean Jjimjilbang

A *jjimjilbang* is a traditional Korean bathhouse that serves as a communal space for bathing, relaxation, and socializing. The jjimjilbang offers a range of facilities, including gender-segregated hot baths, various types of saunas, and steam rooms where therapeutic minerals are sometimes provided. These facilities, reputed for health benefits, are an integral part of Korean wellness culture. In addition to bathing areas, jjimjilbangs feature gender-integrated communal resting areas . These areas are equipped with heated floors, and visitors often wear special uniforms provided by the jjimjilbang to lounge or even sleep on mats. Fitness centers and game rooms are common, and food is also essential to the jjimjilbang experience.

### Steam Room

A steam room is a heated room filled with water vapor to create a high-humidity environment. It is typically maintained at temperatures between 43°C and 49°C (110°F and 120°F). A steam generator boils water and releases steam into the room, creating a humidity level close to 100%. The high humidity of the steam room prevents the body's capacity for evaporative cooling, which limits exposure time.

### Infrared Sauna

An infrared sauna uses infrared heaters to emit infrared light absorbed by the skin's surface. Unlike traditional saunas that heat the air, infrared saunas directly warm the body. They typically operate at a lower temperature (120-140°F or 49-60°C) compared to traditional saunas (150-180°F or 66-82°C). Many infrared saunas are designed for home use, making them convenient for those who want to enjoy sauna benefits without visiting a spa or gym.

### Conclusion

The sauna's role in culture has transitioned from a daily necessity to primarily a luxury or health and wellness activity enjoyed in gyms and spas and as a leisure activity at holiday resorts. But, as awareness grows about the health benefits of sauna therapy, coupled with an increasing focus on holistic wellness, saunas are poised to become a more mainstream method of self-care that will continue to evolve and adapt to the needs of future generations.

# PART TWO

## HEAT, HEALTH, AND HEALING: SAUNA PRACTICE TO PREVENT, HALT, AND REVERSE DISEASE PROCESSES

Before the advent of civilization, some 12,000 years ago, humans lived in a constant state of physical exertion in order to survive. Activities such as hunting, gathering food, and constructing shelters demanded high energy expenditure. Combined with continuous exposure to natural elements like sun, wind, and rain, these pursuits regularly pushed the human body to its physical limits. This lifestyle kept our ancestors in peak physical conditioning, their bodies constantly adapting to environmental challenges and strenuous tasks.

In contrast, we spend much less energy today owing to increasingly sedentary lifestyles, mechanization, and technological advancements. Climate technologies enable us to shield ourselves from temperature extremes. The shift from an active outdoor lifestyle to a more sedentary, indoor one has had profound implications for human physiology and health, potentially impacting metabolic functions and thermoregulatory adaptations.

Today's challenge is to mindfully create a lifestyle that mimics the optimal environmental conditions of our prehistoric evolutionary ancestors. Against this backdrop of the modern-day health challenge, sauna therapy is emerging as a powerful tool for correcting bodily dysfunction and promoting overall well-being. By subjecting the body to controlled doses of heat stress, sauna therapy can help stimulate the body's natural healing mechanisms and improve how our bodies function at every level.

In this section, we explore the therapeutic effects of heat stress on the body. We first examine the effects of heat stress at the molecular and cellular levels. We then expand our investigation to explore the therapeutic effects of heat throughout the body's intricate and interrelated organ systems.

This section provides insight into why sauna therapy can serve as a holistic, integrated approach to correcting a wide range of bodily disorders that are prevalent, and in some cases epidemic, in today's society. By addressing the root causes of these disorders rather than merely treating the symptoms, sauna therapy offers a promising avenue for restoring balance and promoting optimal health.

# 4. Enhancing Molecular and Cellular Function

The *heat shock response* (HSR) is the cellular defense mechanism triggered by heat stress. It activates several cellular-level processes that trigger a cascade of beneficial adaptations. This section describes these adaptive responses to heat stress, exploring the intricate interplay between heat shock protein (HSP) expression, autophagy, mitochondrial function, and oxidative stress management in regular sauna use.

### Heat Shock Proteins

Proteins are large, complex molecules made up of amino acids that perform a wide variety of essential functions in living organisms, including catalyzing biochemical reactions, providing structural support, and facilitating cell signaling and communication. Proteins are nature's workhorses that carry out the cells' functions necessary for life.

Heat shock proteins (HSPs) are a group of proteins responsible for caring for other proteins in the cells so they can do their work. HSPs keep proteins in order by repairing or helping to eliminate them. Because proteins are potentially damaged by heat stress, HSPs are critical in helping cells cope with stress. By maintaining protein homeostasis, or a state of balance, HSPs contribute to cellular resilience and recovery from stressful conditions.

HSPs are highly conserved across different species and found in the cells of all forms of life, indicating their essential role in cellular protection and survival. In addition to responding to heat, they are also upregulated in response to other stressors, such as infection, inflammation, and exposure to toxins.

The heat stress experienced during sauna sessions triggers a marked increase in HSP expression, leading to a number of adaptive responses:

### Protein folding

HSPs act as molecular chaperones, assisting in the proper folding of proteins. Proteins need to be folded into specific shapes to function correctly. HSPs guide this process, ensuring proteins achieve and maintain their correct configurations.

### Cell protection during stress

During stressful conditions such as heat exposure, toxins, or physical injury, HSPs protect cellular proteins from damage. They shield proteins from unfolding and aggregation, maintaining cellular function.

### Protein quality control

HSPs are critical in identifying misfolded or damaged proteins. They prevent these defective proteins from clumping together and tag them for degradation. This quality control mechanism is vital for cellular health and function.

### Cell signaling regulation

HSPs are involved in cell signaling pathways, ensuring proper cell communication. They interact with proteins involved in these pathways, facilitating accurate signal transmission.

### Systemic thermoregulation

HSPs contribute to the systemic thermoregulatory response at the organism level by protecting vital organs and tissues from heat damage. This process is essential in endothermic animals (e.g., mammals and birds), which maintain a constant body temperature through metabolic heat production and other physiological mechanisms. HSPs help maintain a stable internal body temperature by protecting cells from heat-induced damage and supporting cellular homeostasis. HSPs regulate the hypothalamic-pituitary-adrenal (HPA) axis, which controls stress response, metabolism, and immune function.

### Oxidative Stress

Oxidative stress is a condition that occurs when there is an imbalance between the production of free radicals, particularly Reactive Oxygen Species (ROS), or oxygen-containing free radicals, and the body's ability to neutralize them with antioxidants. ROS and other free radicals are unstable molecules with unpaired electrons, making them highly reactive.

At the molecular level, these unpaired electrons create an imbalance in the atom's outermost shell, causing the ROS or free radical to seek stability by "stealing" an electron from nearby molecules. This electron theft can trigger a chain reaction, as the molecule that lost an electron becomes a new free radical, potentially damaging cellular components like proteins, lipids, and DNA. ROS, which includes molecules such as superoxide, hydrogen peroxide, and hydroxyl radicals, are especially significant in this process as they are continuously produced in cells as byproducts of normal oxygen metabolism and can rapidly accumulate under certain conditions.

Antioxidants are molecules that neutralize free radicals and reactive oxygen species. They help prevent or reduce oxidative stress by donating electrons to stabilize these reactive molecules without becoming unstable themselves, thus protecting cellular components from damage.

Oxidative stress dysregulation occurs when there's an imbalance between the production of free radicals and the body's ability to neutralize them with antioxidants, leading to cellular damage and potential health issues such as:

- Chronic inflammation
- Accelerated aging
- Cardiovascular disease
- Neurodegenerative disorders (e.g., Alzheimer's and Parkinson's diseases)
- Cancer
- Diabetes
- Autoimmune disorders

Maintaining a balance between free radicals and antioxidants is crucial for overall health and disease prevention. While excessive oxidative stress can be detrimental to cellular health, the moderate oxidative stress induced by sauna use can paradoxically strengthen the body's antioxidant defenses:

- Controlled ROS production: Sauna heat stress induces a mild increase in the production of reactive oxygen species (ROS). This controlled oxidative challenge activates the cell's antioxidant defense mechanisms.
- Antioxidant system upregulation: Regular sauna use leads to the upregulation of endogenous or internal antioxidant systems. This response includes increased levels of key antioxidant enzymes such as superoxide dismutase (SOD), catalase, and elevated glutathione levels. These adaptations enhance the body's capacity to neutralize free radicals and manage oxidative stress more effectively.

### Mitochondrial Dynamics

Mitochondria are organelles (specialized structures within cells) that serve as cellular powerhouses, generating energy that sustains life through a number of cellular functions:

#### Energy production

Mitochondria are the primary site of ATP production. ATP, or adenosine triphosphate, is a complex organic molecule that is the primary energy carrier in all living organisms. It plays a crucial role in cellular processes by providing the energy needed for various biological functions. ATP is the cell's energy currency, necessary for numerous cellular processes, including muscle contraction, nerve impulse propagation, and biosynthesis. Mitochondria produce reactive oxygen species (ROS) as byproducts of the electron transport chain (ETC) during aerobic respiration. Reactive oxygen species (ROS) are highly reactive molecules that contain oxygen. These species are free radicals formed as natural byproducts of the normal metabolism of oxygen.

#### Reactive oxygen species (ROS) management

While mitochondria produce reactive oxygen species as byproducts of ATP production, they also have mechanisms to detoxify these ROS. Maintaining a balance between ROS production and detoxification is essential to prevent oxidative stress, damaging cellular components and contributing to aging and disease.

### Metabolic regulation

Mitochondria are involved in various metabolic pathways, including the citric acid cycle (Krebs cycle), fatty acid oxidation, and amino acid metabolism. These pathways are critical for maintaining energy balance and metabolic homeostasis. Efficient mitochondrial function ensures proper glucose and lipid metabolism, which is crucial for maintaining healthy blood sugar and lipid levels. Conditions like obesity, diabetes, and metabolic syndrome are associated with impaired mitochondrial function. Enhancing mitochondrial health can improve metabolic outcomes and reduce the risk of these disorders. Metabolism is discussed in greater depth in Chapter Nine.

### Apoptosis regulation

Mitochondria play a crucial role in apoptosis, the process of programmed cell death. This process is important for removing damaged or dysfunctional cells and maintaining tissue homeostasis. Dysregulation of apoptosis can lead to diseases such as cancer (too little apoptosis) or neurodegenerative diseases (too much apoptosis).

### Calcium homeostasis

Mitochondria help regulate intracellular calcium levels, vital for various cellular processes, including muscle contraction, neurotransmitter release, and cell signaling.

### Mitochondrial biogenesis and dynamics

Forming new mitochondria is essential for adapting to increased energy demands, such as during exercise or stress. PGC-1α is a key regulator of mitochondrial biogenesis. Mitochondria continuously undergo fission (splitting) and fusion (joining), crucial for maintaining mitochondrial function, distribution, and quality control. Disruptions in these processes are associated with various diseases.

### Aging and longevity

Mitochondrial dysfunction is closely linked to the aging process. The accumulation of mitochondrial DNA mutations, reduced ATP production, and increased oxidative stress contribute to the age-related decline in cellular function. Sauna practice and other interventions that improve mitochondrial function (e.g., caloric restriction, exercise, and certain dietary supplements such as NAD+ precursors and antioxidants) are associated with increased lifespan and improved health span.

Exposure to intense heat, such as during a sauna session, can have several beneficial effects on mitochondria. These effects are often related to the cellular stress response and adaptations that enhance mitochondrial function and overall cellular health.

### Enhanced mitochondrial biogenesis

Heat stress can stimulate the production of new mitochondria in cells, a process known as *mitochondrial biogenesis*.

### Mitohormesis

Mild heat stress can induce a beneficial response called *mitohormesis*, where low levels of mitochondrial stress stimulate protective mechanisms that ultimately improve mitochondrial function and resilience.

### Improved mitochondrial function

Regular heat exposure can enhance mitochondrial efficiency and function, improving the efficiency of the electron transport chain, better ATP production, and reducing the production of reactive oxygen species (ROS). Mild heat stress can enhance the efficiency of mitochondrial energy production by activating *sirtuins*, a family of proteins involved in cellular metabolism and longevity. Sirtuins can stimulate mitochondrial function and reduce oxidative stress, improving energy production and cellular health.

### Mitochondrial efficiency

Repeated exposure to the controlled heat stress of sauna sessions acts as a hormetic stimulus, prompting the body to adapt at the cellular level. This adaptation includes enhanced mitochondrial efficiency, allowing these organelles to produce energy more effectively.

### Efficient ATP production

Improved mitochondrial function and increased mitochondrial numbers allow cells to produce adenosine triphosphate (ATP) more efficiently. ATP is the cell's primary energy currency, and its increased availability supports overall cellular health and function.

### Autophagy and Cellular Renewal

Autophagy, a term derived from the Greek words for self-eating, is a crucial cellular process that plays a significant role in the body's response to sauna-induced heat stress. This highly conserved mechanism involves degrading and recycling cellular components, including damaged proteins, organelles, and other cellular debris.

Regular sauna use has been shown to stimulate autophagy, contributing to cellular health and longevity in several ways:

### Cellular Cleaning

Heat stress activates autophagy pathways, prompting cells to clear out damaged or dysfunctional components. This "housekeeping" process helps maintain cellular integrity and function.

### Stress resistance

By removing damaged cellular components, autophagy enhances the cell's ability to withstand various forms of stress, including oxidative stress and inflammation.

### Longevity promotion

Efficient autophagy is associated with increased lifespan in various organisms. By regularly inducing autophagy, sauna use may contribute to overall longevity.

### Metabolic regulation

Autophagy plays a role in metabolic homeostasis, influencing glucose metabolism and lipid breakdown processes.

### Neuroprotection

Autophagy helps clear protein aggregates associated with neurodegenerative diseases in the brain, potentially offering neuroprotective benefits.

As cells learn to cope with the controlled stress of heat exposure, they become more efficient at initiating autophagy, potentially leading to improved cellular function and resilience over time.

## Integrative Cellular Response to Sauna Therapy

The cellular processes influenced by sauna use do not operate in isolation but form an intricate network of adaptive responses:

### Hormetic adaptation

The mild stress induced by sauna sessions activates a hormetic response, a beneficial adaptation to mild stress wherein the body becomes more resilient. This adaptation encompasses autophagy, improved mitochondrial function, enhanced antioxidant defenses, and increased HSP expression.

### Cellular resilience

The combined effects of upregulated antioxidant systems and increased HSP levels result in cells that are more resistant to various forms of stress, including heat. This enhanced resilience improves overall health, reduces inflammation, and better manages oxidative stress.

### Performance and recovery

For individuals engaged in regular physical activity, the cellular adaptations induced by sauna use can translate into improved muscle recovery and enhanced performance due to enhanced mitochondrial function and reduced oxidative damage facilitated by elevated HSP levels.

The cellular mechanisms that sauna therapy activates have far-reaching health and well-being implications. Regular sauna use has been associated with improved cardiovascular function, enhanced detoxification processes, boosted immune function, and positive effects on mental health. These benefits can be traced back to the adaptive responses at the cellular level, where mitochondrial function is optimized, oxidative stress is better managed, and heat shock proteins offer enhanced cellular protection.

### Conclusion

In summary, the controlled heat stress from sauna use initiates a series of beneficial cellular-level adaptations that work in concert to enhance overall health and resilience. Regular heat exposure can lead to numerous beneficial adaptations in the body through the stimulation of heat shock proteins, regulation of oxidative stress, and enhancement of mitochondrial function and autophagy. The cellular and molecular changes induced by heat stress contribute to improved heat acclimatization, better physical functioning, and potentially increased lifespan. By understanding these biological responses to heat, we can appreciate the sauna as a powerful holistic therapeutic practice with far-reaching benefits.

# 5. Enhancing Brain and Nervous System Functions

The nervous system is a complex network of cells and tissues that serves as the body's leading communication and control center. It consists of the brain, spinal cord, and a vast network of nerves that extend throughout the body. The nervous system's primary functions include receiving and processing sensory information from the environment and the body's internal organs, initiating and coordinating motor responses, regulating bodily functions such as heart rate, breathing, and digestion, and enabling cognitive functions like thinking, learning, memory, and emotions. The nervous system transmits electrical and chemical signals between neurons, allowing rapid communication and response to stimuli, ensuring the body functions effectively and maintains homeostasis.

Heat stress can have a number of positive effects on nervous system functions, described below.

**Balance the Stress Response**

The human body's stress response is a complex, automatic physiological reaction to perceived threats or challenges. When faced with stress, our body activates two key systems: the sympathetic nervous system and the hypothalamic-pituitary-adrenal (HPA) axis. The sympathetic nervous system, part of our autonomic nervous system, triggers the "fight or flight" response. It rapidly prepares the body for action by increasing heart rate, dilating pupils, raising blood pressure, and diverting blood flow to muscles and the brain. It also suppresses digestion and releases glucose for quick energy. The HPA axis is a complex neuroendocrine system that works in tandem with the sympathetic nervous system. It involves the hypothalamus in the brain, the pituitary gland at the brain's base, and the adrenal glands atop the kidneys.

The CRH (Corticotropin-Releasing Hormone) system initiates the HPA axis response and the body's initial response to stress. When we encounter a stressor, the hypothalamus in our brain releases CRH, which sets off a chain reaction. This hormone travels to the pituitary gland, prompting it to release another hormone called ACTH, Adrenocorticotropic Hormone. ACTH then signals the adrenal glands to produce cortisol, our primary stress hormone, which helps regulate metabolism, immune function, and the body's overall stress response. This cascade helps prepare our body to handle stress, affecting everything from energy levels to immune function. However, if constantly activated due to chronic stress, the CRH system can become overworked, potentially leading to various health issues.

Chronic stress can lead to dysregulation of this system, often resulting in an imbalance favoring sympathetic dominance over parasympathetic activity and contributing to various stress-related disorders, including anxiety, depression, and post-traumatic stress disorder (PTSD).

Adrenal dysregulation is an example of the body's response to chronic stress. Adrenal dysregulation occurs when the adrenal glands, responsible for producing stress hormones such as cortisol and adrenaline, become overworked and unable to regulate their output effectively. Dysregulation can lead to a wide range of symptoms, including fatigue, anxiety, migraines, depression and other mood imbalances, and difficulty sleeping, as well as conditions such as fibromyalgia and irritable bowel syndrome. Chronic stress, which is often a precursor to adrenal dysregulation, can also have a significant impact on overall health and well-being.

A balanced stress response is crucial for overall health and well-being. When functioning optimally, the body reacts appropriately to acute stressors and efficiently returns to equilibrium. This balance supports immune function, cognitive performance, cardiovascular health, metabolism, sleep regulation, and mood stability.

When the stress response is normalized, balance is restored to the autonomic nervous system by reducing excessive cortisol production and improving the regulation of neurotransmitters like norepinephrine. By inducing a controlled, acute stress response, sauna use may help reduce chronic stress, restore autonomic balance, improve stress resilience, and potentially enhance HPA axis function over time, ultimately contributing to improved overall health and well-being.

### *Stress and the social world*

Our nervous systems develop through our social interactions within the cultural environment. Just as our bodies need food, our emotional well-being depends on healthy relationships. When we're in unhealthy relationships, chronic stress prevents the body from returning to its normal, balanced state. Our stress response is triggered by how we perceive threats in our environment. Chronic, prolonged stress response activation ultimately leads to dysregulation of the nervous system. Anxiety becomes a dominant force, shaping how we perceive and react to the world around us. To heal, we need to create new neural pathways associated with calmness and relaxation.

By developing greater awareness and control over our thought patterns, we can learn to interpret situations differently. This allows us to manage our emotional reactions better and reduce unnecessary stress responses.

Enduring high temperatures in the sauna is a practice in stress resilience. In my experience, daily 90-minute sauna sessions, typically in the evening, have been particularly effective in balancing my stress hormones. The session lowers my cortisol levels, which are abnormally high in the morning and spike throughout the day instead of following a healthy decline. Figure 5-1 shows the dramatic effect of a 90-minute sauna session in lowering my cortisol levels. Even though my nighttime levels are higher than average, I can now sleep. Before discovering sauna therapy, I couldn't sleep because I couldn't relax my body, and I developed a dependence on benzodiazepines, sleep medications, and the urge to use alcohol as a coping mechanism, all of which contributed to my deteriorating health.

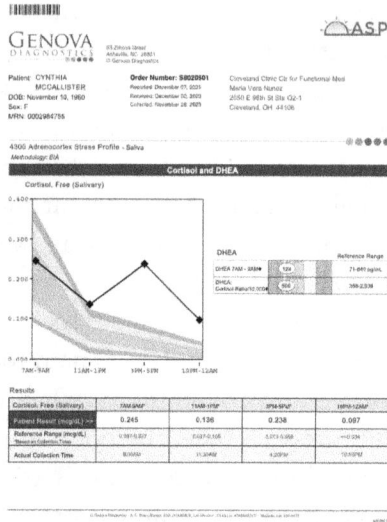

*Figure 6-1: Day-long Cortisol Test*

## Stimulate the Vague Nerve

The vagus nerve, also known as the tenth cranial nerve (CN X), plays a crucial role in enhancing the activity of the parasympathetic nervous system and maintaining a balance between the sympathetic and parasympathetic nervous systems, which is essential for overall autonomic health. This important nerve regulates various body functions, including heart rate, blood pressure, digestion, and stress response. It also supports mental health, immune function, and respiratory health and is a key component of the gut-brain axis. When the vagus nerve functions optimally, it enhances parasympathetic activity, counteracts sympathetic dominance, and promotes overall well-being.

Common symptoms of vagus nerve dysregulation include digestive issues, heart rate irregularities, difficulty swallowing, anxiety, depression, chronic fatigue, and heightened stress responses. Vagus Nerve Stimulation (VNS) is an emerging intervention used to treat epilepsy and treatment-resistant depression.

Heat exposure from sauna use can naturally stimulate the vagus nerve through various physiological mechanisms, including muscle relaxation, improved blood circulation, reduced inflammation, and enhanced heart rate variability. This stimulation can increase vagal tone, which is associated with a more resilient stress response system and better overall health.

### Regulate the Neurotransmitter System

Heat stress significantly influences the brain's neurotransmitter systems, affecting mood, cognition, and neurological function. It primarily impacts the release and activity of key neurotransmitters such as serotonin, dopamine, norepinephrine, glutamate, and GABA (gamma-aminobutyric acid). These neurotransmitters play crucial roles in brain function and behavior.

Serotonin regulates mood, sleep, appetite, and pain sensation and is often associated with feelings of well-being and happiness. Dopamine is involved in reward, motivation, pleasure, and motor control and is key in reinforcing behaviors. Norepinephrine influences alertness, attention, and the body's fight-or-flight response, enhancing focus and energy. Glutamate is the primary excitatory neurotransmitter, crucial for learning, memory, and synaptic plasticity. As the main inhibitory neurotransmitter, GABA reduces neuronal excitability, promoting relaxation and reducing anxiety.

These neurotransmitters work in concert to maintain balance in brain function, influencing various aspects of cognition, emotion, and behavior. These changes can lead to altered mood states, shifts in motivation and reward processing, and modifications in alertness, attention, and stress responses.

Over time, regular exposure to heat stress from the sauna may lead to adaptive changes in these neurotransmitter systems, potentially enhancing stress resilience and overall mental well-being.

### Increase Nitric Oxide Production

Nitric oxide is a signaling molecule that transmits information between cells. Nitric oxide production significantly enhances the body's stress response through multiple mechanisms. As a potent vasodilator, it improves blood flow and helps regulate blood pressure, counteracting the effects of stress hormones. Nitric oxide also acts as a neurotransmitter, modulating the release of other stress-related neurotransmitters in the brain. Its anti-inflammatory properties help mitigate stress-induced inflammation, while its role in endothelial and immune function supports overall physiological resilience. Increased nitric oxide production improves circulation, reduces inflammation, and supports various bodily systems, helping the body maintain balance and respond more effectively to stressors, potentially mitigating the negative impacts of acute and chronic stress. Exposure to heat stress from the sauna potentially boosts nitric oxide production.

**Improve Sleep**

Sleep is one of the most critical factors for overall health and well-being. During sleep, the body repairs itself, memories are consolidated in the brain, and important hormones that regulate everything from appetite to immune function are released. Chronic insufficient sleep has been linked to an increased risk of obesity, diabetes, heart disease, depression, and cognitive impairment. Unfortunately, many people struggle to get enough high-quality sleep regularly. Stress, medical conditions, sleep disorders, and poor sleep hygiene can all impair the ability to fall asleep and stay asleep through the night.

Research has shown that sauna use, especially in the evening, can significantly improve sleep quality and help treat insomnia symptoms. Here are some of the key ways sauna practice positively impacts sleep:

*Increases slow-wave sleep*

Studies have found that sauna sessions, especially at night, increase the amount of slow-wave sleep, also known as deep sleep. This is the most physically restorative stage of sleep, when muscles relax, tissues repair, and hormones are released. Spending more time in deep sleep results in feeling more rested and refreshed the next day.

Reduces Sleep Latency: Sleep latency refers to the time it takes to fall asleep after getting into bed. If you often lie awake for a long time before drifting off, you have a long sleep latency. Sauna use has been shown to shorten sleep latency, helping you fall asleep faster. The relaxation effects of the sauna carry over to bedtime.

Improves sleep efficiency: Sleep efficiency is the percentage of time you spend asleep while in bed. Ideally, it should be 85% or higher. Saunas boost sleep efficiency by extending total sleep time and reducing nighttime awakenings and restlessness, meaning more time in bed is spent sleeping.

### Alleviates stress and anxiety

Stress and anxiety are among the most common causes of sleep trouble. By promoting deep relaxation, saunas help calm the mind and reduce psychological arousal before bed. The wave of relaxation you feel after a sauna session can make it much easier to wind down and clear your head at the end of the day.

### Provides exercise recovery

For people who exercise later in the day or evening, post-workout muscle soreness and central nervous system activation can make it hard to fall asleep. Taking a sauna after training accelerates recovery and relaxes the body, counteracting the stimulating effects of nighttime exercise.

### Positively influences the circadian rhythm

The circadian rhythm is a natural, internal process that regulates various physiological functions in living organisms, including the sleep-wake cycle, hormone production, body temperature, and metabolism. Exposure to high temperatures in a sauna can mimic the body's natural temperature fluctuations throughout the day. The circadian rhythm is closely tied to these temperature changes, with body temperature dropping at night and rising during the day. Sauna sessions can help reinforce this pattern.

### Stimulates melatonin production

Sauna use may increase melatonin production, a hormone that regulates the sleep-wake cycle. Melatonin levels naturally rise in the evening, promoting sleep, and decrease in the morning, promoting wakefulness. Regular sauna sessions can help maintain a healthy melatonin balance.

To maximize the sleep benefits, aim to sauna bathe at least 1-2 hours before your target bedtime to give your body time to cool down before sleep. Combine your sauna habit with other healthy sleep tips like keeping a consistent sleep schedule, avoiding late caffeine, and creating a dark, quiet, cool sleeping environment.

**Relieve Symptoms of Anxiety and Depression**

Sauna therapy has been shown to positively impact a range of chronic stress-related conditions, including anxiety, depression, and chronic fatigue syndrome. By promoting relaxation, reducing inflammation, and normalizing the stress response, sauna therapy can help alleviate the symptoms of these conditions and improve overall quality of life. Heat exposure can also lead to relaxation and an improved sense of well-being.

**Relieve Symptoms of Post-traumatic Stress Disorder**

Treating Post-Traumatic Stress Disorder (PTSD) effectively involves addressing a complex web of bodily dysregulations that occur in response to trauma. At its core, PTSD disrupts the body's stress response system, primarily affecting the autonomic nervous system and the hypothalamic-pituitary-adrenal (HPA) axis. This disruption leads to imbalances in stress hormones like cortisol and alters the functioning of key neurotransmitters such as serotonin, norepinephrine, and dopamine.

Beyond these primary systems, PTSD also impacts brain structures like the amygdala and prefrontal cortex, leading to heightened fear responses and difficulties in emotional regulation. Additionally, it affects sleep patterns, the immune system, and the gut-brain axis.

Addressing PTSD requires a holistic approach that aims to restore balance to these interconnected systems, often combining psychological therapies with physiological interventions to help the body and mind process and integrate the traumatic experience.

Sauna practice is emerging as a promising approach to PTSD treatment by helping reduce stress by lowering cortisol levels, improving sleep quality, increasing neuroplasticity by stimulating BDNF production, and regulating the autonomic nervous system. Additionally, saunas trigger endorphin release, promote mindfulness, and foster social connections in group settings.

**Improve Overall Brain Health and Cognitive Function**

Emerging research suggests that regular sauna bathing may significantly benefit brain health and cognitive function. Cognitive function refers to the brain's ability to process, store, retrieve, and manipulate information. It encompasses a wide range of mental processes that enable us to perceive, learn, remember, reason, and interact with our environment. These processes include attention, memory, language, problem-solving, decision-making, and executive functions such as planning and organizing. Cognitive function is crucial for everyday tasks, from simple activities like recognizing faces and following conversations to complex problem-solving and creative thinking. It forms the basis of our ability to acquire knowledge, adapt to new situations, and navigate social interactions. The health and efficiency of our cognitive functions play a significant role in determining our overall mental performance, quality of life, and ability to function independently.

Sauna use may improve cognitive function through several interrelated mechanisms.

### Improved circulation

First, by enhancing blood flow to the brain, sauna use may help remove metabolic waste products and toxins from the brain more efficiently and ensure better oxygen and nutrient delivery to neural tissues, promoting a healthier brain environment.

### Improved heat shock protein production

Heat shock proteins (HSPs) play a crucial role in protecting brain cells from damage and facilitating clearance of misfolded proteins, such as amyloid-beta, which is strongly associated with developing diseases such as Parkinson's and Alzheimer's. By inducing the production of HSPs, sauna use may help prevent the accumulation of neurotoxic proteins and maintain brain cell integrity.

### Improved mitochondrial function

Neurons are highly dependent on mitochondrial function for energy production. HSR helps maintain mitochondrial integrity and function. Since neurons become more tolerant to subsequent stressors after an initial heat shock, this preconditioning effect can improve their survival during stressful conditions.

### Increased production of antioxidants and anti-inflammatory compounds

Regular sauna use can help prevent neurodegenerative diseases and the accumulation of amyloid tissue by activating cellular defense mechanisms and producing antioxidants and anti-inflammatory compounds that shield brain cells from oxidative stress and inflammation.

### Increased production of brain-derived neurotrophic factor

Brain-derived neurotrophic factor (BDNF) is a protein that supports brain cells' growth, survival, and differentiation. Studies have shown that sauna exposure can increase BDNF levels, suggesting that regular sauna use may help protect against age-related cognitive decline and support the brain's ability to adapt and regenerate.

### Stress reduction

Regular sauna sessions can help alleviate the negative effects of chronic stress on the body by promoting relaxation, lowering cortisol levels, and increasing the production of endorphins. These improvements, in turn, can lead to improved mood, better sleep, and enhanced immune function.

### Neurogenesis

Sauna use may stimulate neurogenesis, the growth of new brain cells, and increase levels of norepinephrine, a neurotransmitter that enhances focus and attention. The heat stress experienced during sauna sessions can trigger a hormesis effect that may enhance cognitive resilience. Improved sleep quality, often reported by regular sauna users, can also indirectly boost cognitive performance through better memory consolidation and overall brain restoration.

### Improved sleep

The relaxation and stress-reducing effects of sauna bathing can indirectly support brain health by promoting better sleep. Adequate sleep is essential for the brain's ability to clear metabolic waste products through the glymphatic system. This unique waste clearance pathway is most active during sleep, making it crucial for maintaining a healthy brain environment. Regular sauna use may enhance the brain's natural cleansing processes and reduce the risk of neurotoxic buildup by improving sleep quality.

### Relieve Psychotic Symptoms

Psychotic disorders, such as schizophrenia, are characterized by a range of symptoms, including delusions, hallucinations, and disordered thinking. Sauna therapy has shown promising results in reducing the severity of psychotic symptoms.

The mechanisms behind the therapeutic effects of sauna heat exposure on psychotic symptoms are believed to be multifaceted.

Heat exposure leads to vasodilation, the widening of blood vessels, and improving circulation and oxygenation throughout the body and brain, probably contributing to a reduction in the intensity and frequency of psychotic symptoms. Another theory suggests that endorphin release during intense heat exposure may help to alleviate the negative symptoms of psychosis, such as apathy, lack of motivation, and social withdrawal. Endorphins are the body's natural "feel-good" chemicals and support a sense of well-being and relaxation. The sauna environment encourages focusing on the present moment and bodily sensations, which can be a form of mindfulness practice. Mindfulness has been shown to reduce stress and improve mental health.

Another mechanism behind the therapeutic effects of sauna heat exposure on psychotic symptoms involves the modulation of neurotransmitters in the brain. Studies have shown that heat stress influences levels of neurotransmitters such as serotonin, dopamine, and norepinephrine, which play a role in the development and maintenance of psychotic disorders. By altering the balance of these neurotransmitters, sauna therapy may help to normalize brain function and reduce the severity of psychotic symptoms.

Individuals with psychotic disorders, such as schizophrenia, often experience significant sleep disturbances, including insomnia, irregular sleep patterns, and disrupted REM sleep. These sleep issues can exacerbate psychotic symptoms, leading to a worsening of hallucinations, delusions, and cognitive impairments. Poor sleep quality affects brain function and emotional regulation, potentially triggering or intensifying psychotic symptoms. Sauna use, especially in the evening, can promote relaxation and enhance sleep quality.

Psychotic disorders are closely linked to social dysfunction, significantly impacting individuals' ability to engage in and maintain social relationships and activities. Symptoms like delusions, hallucinations, and disorganized thinking impair social interactions, leading to difficulties in understanding social cues and communicating effectively. These impairments often result in social isolation, reduced social networks, and challenges maintaining employment or education. Sauna bathing is often a social activity, providing opportunities for social interaction and support, which are important for mental health and recovery from psychotic disorders.

A study conducted by researchers in Finland investigated the effects of regular sauna bathing on individuals with schizophrenia (Laukkanen, Laukkanen, & Kunutsor, 2018). The participants engaged in sauna sessions three times a week for four weeks, each lasting 15 minutes at 80-90°C (176-194°F). The results showed a significant decrease in the severity of both positive symptoms (such as hallucinations and delusions) and negative symptoms (such as emotional flatness and social withdrawal) among the participants. The researchers hypothesized that the improvement in symptoms could be attributed to the sauna's ability to reduce stress, improve sleep quality, and promote a sense of well-being.

**My Nervous System Response**

Heat therapy has enabled me to largely resolve nervous system dysregulation, which was extensive. Given my genetic predisposition to neurological disorders—my sister lost her battle with mental illness, and my mother died from a stroke due to cerebral amyloid angiopathy—finding an effective treatment was crucial for me.

The combined physical and mental benefits of sauna sessions, in addition to greater insight into unhealthy self-perceptions and maladaptive patterns in my relationships through ongoing therapy, have led to a significant recovery. My heart rate is normal, sleep has improved, anxiety has decreased, mood swings have stabilized, I'm no longer depressed, and cognitive function has sharpened, among other improvements too lengthy to mention. I can now control the symptoms of PTSD. These benefits have resulted in a quality of life I previously thought unattainable.

**Conclusion**

In conclusion, heat stress from sauna use offers numerous potential benefits for nervous system function and overall health. Regular sauna sessions may help balance the body's stress response, stimulate the vagus nerve, regulate neurotransmitter systems, increase nitric oxide production, and improve sleep quality. These effects can potentially alleviate symptoms of anxiety, depression, PTSD, and even psychotic disorders. Furthermore, sauna use may enhance cognitive function and brain health by improving circulation, stimulating the production of protective proteins, and promoting neuroplasticity. While more research is needed to fully understand the mechanisms and optimal protocols, the evidence suggests that incorporating regular sauna sessions into one's routine could be a valuable strategy for supporting nervous system health and overall well-being. As always, individuals should consult with healthcare professionals before beginning any new health regimen, especially those with pre-existing conditions.

# 6. Enhancing Circulatory System Functions

Cardiovascular disease (CVD) is a leading cause of death worldwide, affecting millions of individuals each year. While lifestyle modifications such as diet and exercise are well-known strategies for reducing the risk of CVD, emerging research suggests that regular sauna bathing may also significantly mitigate the effects of this condition.

Several observational studies have provided evidence for the cardiovascular benefits of sauna bathing. For example, a large prospective study conducted in Finland found that men who engaged in sauna bathing 4-7 times per week had a 50% lower risk of fatal CVD compared to those who used the sauna only once per week. Another study demonstrated that regular sauna use was associated with a reduced risk of sudden cardiac death, a major cause of mortality in individuals with CVD.

In this chapter, we explore how sauna bathing may help mitigate the effects of CVD. As previously discussed, heat stress from sauna bathing stimulates the production of heat shock proteins. These proteins help protect the heart and blood vessels from damage and improve their function. Several other benefits of sauna bathing help mitigate the effects of CVD.

### Improve Endothelial Function

The heat stress induced by sauna bathing has been shown to improve endothelial function, which is critical for maintaining healthy blood vessels. Endothelial function refers to the health and performance of the endothelium, a thin cell layer lining blood vessels. It regulates blood flow, blood pressure, and clotting, acts as a barrier, and is involved in inflammation and new blood vessel formation. Enhanced endothelial function can help prevent the development of atherosclerosis, a major contributor to CVD. Healthy endothelial function is essential for cardiovascular health, while impairment is linked to atherosclerosis, hypertension, and diabetes.

### Reduce Blood Pressure

Regular sauna bathing has been shown to reduce blood pressure. Studies have shown that regular sauna bathing can have long-term benefits for blood pressure management and result in a lower risk of developing hypertension compared to those who do not. This effect is thought to be mediated by several factors:

### *Vasodilation and improved circulation*

When exposed to high temperatures in a sauna, the body's blood vessels dilate, allowing for increased blood flow. This vasodilation process reduces the resistance to blood flow, which in turn lowers blood pressure. The improved circulation also helps deliver oxygen and nutrients more efficiently to various body parts, promoting better overall health.

### *Reduction in stress hormones*

Stress significantly contributes to high blood pressure. Sauna bathing has been found to reduce levels of stress hormones such as cortisol and norepinephrine. As these hormones decrease, the body becomes more relaxed, which can help lower blood pressure.

Increased Sweating and Fluid Loss: Sweating during sauna sessions leads to fluid loss, which can temporarily lower blood pressure. While this effect is short-lived, regular sauna use can help maintain a healthy fluid balance, improving blood pressure regulation.

### *Improved endothelial function*

Improved endothelial function, described above, allows the blood vessels to relax and dilate more effectively, leading to better blood pressure control.

**Increase Cardiac Output and Maximal Oxygen Uptake (VO2 max)**

Sauna bathing can increase cardiac output, which is the amount of blood pumped by the heart per minute. Increased cardiac output means more blood is circulated through the body per minute. Since blood carries oxygen (bound to hemoglobin in red blood cells), more blood flow results in more oxygen being transported throughout the body. The primary purpose of circulating more blood is to meet the increased oxygen demands of tissues. When the heart rate goes up, it is typically a response to the body's need for more energy and oxygen. Thus, a higher heart rate, within an optimal range, can effectively increase the circulation of blood and oxygen delivery to where it is needed most. This adaptation is particularly crucial during periods of physical activity or stress when the body's oxygen and nutrient demands are higher.

Sauna bathing can also increase the maximal oxygen uptake (VO2 max), the maximum rate at which the body can consume oxygen during intense exercise. VO2 max is a key indicator of cardiovascular fitness and aerobic endurance. Increased oxygen intake can have several positive effects on health and overall well-being, as explained below.

*Improved energy levels and cognitive function*

Oxygen is crucial for producing energy in the form of adenosine triphosphate (ATP). With higher oxygen levels, your body can produce more energy efficiently, leading to improved mental clarity, focus, and cognitive functions.

*Enhanced exercise performance*

Increasing oxygen intake can improve athletic performance. It helps in faster oxygen delivery to muscles, which is beneficial during intense workouts or sports, reducing the feeling of fatigue and improving endurance.

*Better immune system function*

Adequate oxygen levels can support the immune system. They aid in the function of white blood cells, which use oxygen to help fight off bacteria and viruses, leading to a reduced risk of infections and a stronger immune response.

### Stress reduction

Increasing oxygen intake can have a calming effect on the mind and body by helping reduce stress and promoting relaxation by lowering the levels of stress hormones in the body.

### Detoxification

Oxygen is vital for the body's metabolic processes, including the detoxification process. It helps to break down toxins and waste products, making it easier for the body to remove them.

### Improved healing and recovery

Increased oxygen levels can accelerate the healing process, particularly in tissues and cells that have been damaged due to injury or surgery. Oxygen helps in cell regeneration and is often used in medical treatments to enhance recovery.

### Improved cardiovascular health

Higher oxygen intake can improve heart function and the efficiency of blood circulation, leading to better oxygenation of the entire body, which benefits cardiovascular health. This adaptation may help improve overall cardiovascular efficiency and reduce the workload on the heart.

### Reduced inflammation

Chronic inflammation is a key driver of CVD, and sauna bathing has been shown to reduce levels of inflammatory markers such as C-reactive protein (CRP). Elevated CRP levels can be associated with an increased risk of cardiovascular diseases, as inflammation plays a role in the development of atherosclerosis. By calming inflammation, regular sauna use may help slow the progression of CVD. See this chapter's section on the Immune System to learn more about CRP. The potential of sauna practice to improve immune system function is discussed in Chapter Ten.

### Lower Heart Rate and Improve Heart Rate Recovery

Mortality risk is closely associated with heart rate, particularly resting heart rate (RHR). Studies have shown that higher RHR correlates with increased risks of death from various causes, including cardiovascular diseases and cancers (Seviiri et al., 2023). Significant increases in RHR over time are linked to even higher mortality rates, emphasizing the importance of RHR monitoring for early intervention. Long-term research has also demonstrated that elevated RHR is associated with lower physical fitness and higher levels of various health risk factors, with individuals having RHR above 90 bpm facing a threefold increase in mortality risk compared to those with RHR below 50 bpm (Jensen et al., 2013).

Sauna practice can powerfully lower heart rate and improve heart rate recovery. The sauna's heat causes blood vessels to dilate, increasing blood flow and circulation throughout the body. As a result, the heart rate increases to accommodate the increased demand for blood flow to the skin for cooling. This process is similar to what happens during moderate-intensity exercise. As the heart strengthens, it becomes more efficient at pumping blood, leading to a lower resting heart rate over time. A lower resting heart rate is generally associated with better cardiovascular fitness and a reduced risk of heart disease. Studies have shown frequent sauna users tend to have lower resting heart rates than non-users.

In addition to lowering resting heart rate, sauna bathing can improve *heart rate recovery*. Heart rate recovery refers to how quickly your heart rate returns to its resting level after physical activity or stress. A faster heart rate recovery indicates good cardiovascular health and fitness. After a sauna session, the heart rate gradually decreases as the body cools down. Over time, with consistent sauna use, the heart becomes more efficient at recovering from the heat stress, leading to improved heart rate recovery.

**Improve Autonomic Function**

Sauna bathing has been associated with improved *heart rate variability* (HRV), a marker of autonomic function. A well-functioning autonomic nervous system is essential for maintaining cardiovascular health and reducing the risk of arrhythmias. Heart rate variability (HRV) is the variation in the time intervals between consecutive heartbeats, known as *interbeat intervals*. It reflects the heart's ability to respond to physiological and environmental stimuli. The autonomic nervous system influences HRV, specifically the balance between the sympathetic nervous system (which accelerates heart rate) and the parasympathetic nervous system (which slows it down).

High HRV generally indicates a healthy, adaptable cardiovascular system, suggesting good autonomic function and resilience to stress.

Conversely, low HRV can be a sign of stress, fatigue, or underlying health issues, and it is often associated with an increased risk of cardiovascular diseases and other health problems. HRV is commonly measured using electrocardiograms (ECGs) or heart rate monitors, and it is used in various fields, including sports science, stress management, and medical diagnostics.

### Conclusion

In conclusion, regular sauna bathing is a promising complementary approach to mitigating cardiovascular disease (CVD) effects. Through improved endothelial function, reduced blood pressure, increased cardiac output and VO2 max, reduced inflammation, and lowered heart rate with improved recovery and enhanced autonomic function, sauna use offers multiple cardiovascular benefits. These effects collectively contribute to better heart health and may reduce the risk of fatal CVD events.

While sauna bathing can provide cardiovascular benefits, it should be seen as a complementary practice to support heart health alongside traditional prevention strategies, such as a balanced diet, regular physical activity, and stress management techniques. As with any lifestyle intervention, consulting with a healthcare professional before incorporating sauna bathing into a health management plan is essential.

### Addendum: Kidney Disease

We offer a brief discussion on the therapeutic effects of sauna use in kidney dialysis patients. The urinary system is responsible for liquid flow that eliminates toxins like urea and heavy metals from the body. Using a sauna can have both benefits and risks for individuals undergoing kidney dialysis. Sweating in the sauna removes waste, potentially reducing the burden on the kidneys. This process, known as dermatodialysis, can support the elimination of wastes that the kidneys usually filter, offering an adjunct to dialysis treatment and improving overall kidney function.

However, there are significant risks associated with sauna use for dialysis patients. Excessive heat can lead to dehydration, hyperthermia, and imbalances in electrolytes, which can be dangerous for individuals with impaired kidney function. It's crucial to use saunas under medical supervision to avoid these complications.

# 7. Enhancing Respiratory System Functions

The respiratory system is a complex network of organs and tissues that facilitates the exchange of oxygen and carbon dioxide between the body and the environment, primarily through breathing.

In recent years, scientific research has shed light on the potential to improve lung capacity and respiratory function with regular sauna use. One of these responses to the rise in body temperature in the sauna is an increase in heart rate and blood flow, which enhances the oxygen delivery and nutrients to the body's organs, including the lungs. The increased heart rate and blood circulation induced by the heat also help to thin the mucus, making it less sticky and easier to remove. Heat can also help loosen mucus and phlegm in the lungs by relaxing the muscles around the airways, making breathing and expelling mucus easier.

Moreover, the deep breathing that naturally occurs during sauna sessions can help to strengthen the respiratory muscles, including the diaphragm and intercostal muscles. As these muscles become stronger, they can more effectively support the lungs in drawing in and expelling air, increasing lung capacity and function over time. A study published in the European Journal of Applied Physiology found that regular sauna bathing can significantly improve lung function and exercise capacity.

The researchers observed that participants who engaged in sauna sessions twice a week for three months experienced a significant increase in vital capacity (the maximum amount of air that can be expelled from the lungs after a deep breath) and forced expiratory volume (the amount of air that can be forcefully exhaled in one second). Additionally, the sweating process aids in eliminating toxins from the body, including those in the respiratory system, thereby reducing inflammation and congestion.

In addition to its direct effects on lung function, sauna bathing can also indirectly support respiratory health by promoting relaxation and reducing stress. The sauna's overall relaxation effect reduces stress and tension, which can also decrease mucus production. Stress compromises the immune system, making individuals more susceptible to respiratory infections. By inducing deep relaxation, sauna sessions can help bolster the body's natural defenses against illness.

### Chronic Obstructive Pulmonary Disease

Sauna bathing may benefit individuals with Chronic Obstructive Pulmonary Disease (COPD) through various mechanisms. The heat and humidity can help loosen mucus and improve airway clearance, potentially easing breathing difficulties. Regular sauna use might reduce systemic inflammation, a key factor in COPD progression while providing cardiovascular benefits and stress reduction. The improved circulation from heat exposure could enhance oxygen delivery to tissues, and the overall experience may strengthen the immune system, potentially reducing the risk of respiratory infections. Additionally, heat stress might improve respiratory muscle function over time. The heat also dilates the airways, allowing for deeper and easier breathing. This helps mobilize and expel mucus more effectively. This effect particularly benefits individuals with respiratory conditions such as asthma, chronic obstructive pulmonary disease (COPD), and bronchitis.

### *COPD case study*

Anecdotally, an acquaintance of mine, who initially suffered from Stage 4 COPD, experienced remarkable improvement after adopting a daily practice of 50 minutes combined time in the sauna and steam room. At the start, he could only walk one city block without needing to rest and could only walk 2,000 steps per day. After eight months of consistent sauna practice, he could maintain a brisk walking pace for 30 minutes and routinely walked 7,000 steps daily, and his condition improved to Stage 3 COPD. Unlike the typical COPD sufferer, he developed heat tolerance quickly, probably because he spent the first 35 years of his life in West Africa, where he recalls harvesting millet in the scorching heat of temperatures above 110. While capillaries may close with frailty, they never completely disappear. Growing up in extreme heat probably contributed to a high capillary density, giving him a unique advantage in adapting to and tolerating the sauna's extreme conditions.

**Conclusion**

In conclusion, regular sauna use offers significant potential benefits for respiratory health and lung function. Through mechanisms such as increased blood flow, improved mucus clearance, strengthened respiratory muscles, and enhanced vital capacity, sauna bathing may contribute to better overall respiratory function. The heat-induced dilation of airways, combined with the relaxation effects, can be particularly beneficial for individuals with respiratory conditions like COPD, asthma, and bronchitis. Additionally, the stress-reducing and immune-boosting effects of sauna use may indirectly support respiratory health by decreasing susceptibility to infections.

While these findings are promising, it's important to note that individuals with pre-existing respiratory conditions should consult their healthcare providers before incorporating sauna use into their wellness routines.

# 8. Enhancing Integumentary (Skin) System Functions

Regular sauna bathing can provide a range of benefits for the body's largest organ—the skin. The skin serves as a protective barrier against external factors such as UV radiation, microorganisms, and physical damage. It plays a crucial role in regulating body temperature through sweat production and dilation or constriction of blood vessels. The skin also helps with sensation, allowing the body to detect pressure, temperature, and pain. Additionally, it synthesizes vitamin D when exposed to sunlight and acts as a waterproof barrier to prevent excessive moisture loss from the body. The skin's appearance can also indicate overall health and well-being. Regular sauna exposure has many benefits for skin quality.

**Improved Circulation and Skin Cell Turnover**

The sauna's heat causes blood vessels in the skin to dilate, increasing circulation and the delivery of oxygen and nutrients to skin cells, improving skin health and sensitivity. This boost in circulation supports the generation of new skin cells and the shedding of old, dead skin cells from the surface. Regular deep cleansing of the pores through sauna bathing helps keep the skin clean, clear, and healthy.

Striking visual evidence that demonstrates the profound effect of prolonged heat exposure on cutaneous blood flow and tissue response is showcased in Figure 8-1. It illustrates what I call "skin dunes"—the distinctive topography visible on the skin's surface after a high-intensity, long-duration sauna session. This picture of the inside of my forearm was taken 15 minutes after a two-hour sauna session. This phenomenon results from the intense vascular activity within the skin's capillaries, causing the surface to bulge and create a landscape reminiscent of sand dunes.

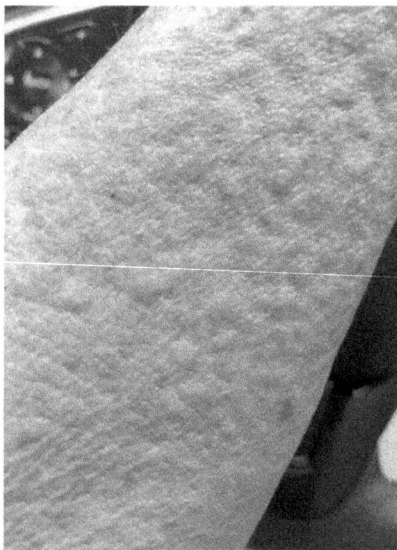

*Figure 8-1: "Skin dunes" on the inside of my arm after a two-hour session in a 160° sauna.*

The outermost layer of skin, the stratum corneum, consists of dead, flattened cells that form a protective barrier. It is constantly shedding and being replaced by newer cells from deeper layers. An excessive buildup of dead cells can trap irritants, bacteria, and moisture against the skin, potentially leading to inflammation and stimulating nerve endings that trigger the itch sensation. The sauna's heat and moisture from sweat help soften this outer layer of skin, making it easier to slough off dead skin afterward. Occasional gentle exfoliation with a loofah or natural bristle brush can effectively slough off dead skin cells, revealing fresher, smoother skin underneath and promoting better circulation.

The result is healthier, more vibrant-looking skin with improved texture and tone.

### Improve Detoxification and Sweating

The human body is constantly exposed to environmental toxins and the foods we consume. These toxins can accumulate in the body over time, leading to various health issues. The sauna can be a powerful tool in supporting detoxification by eliminating these harmful substances from the body through sweating. Sweating during a sauna session opens up and flushes out the pores, releasing dirt, oil, toxins, and other impurities that can clog pores and contribute to acne and blemishes. Sweating can help eliminate a wide range of toxins from the body, including heavy metals, BPA, and PCBs. By removing toxins from the body, detoxification can improve digestion and nutrient absorption, boost immune system function, enhance mental clarity and cognitive function, increase energy levels, promote healthy skin and a clearer complexion, support weight loss efforts, and reduce inflammation and chronic pain.

### Increase Collagen Production

Some research suggests that the heat stress of sauna bathing may stimulate the production of collagen and elastin fibers in the skin. Collagen and elastin are key proteins that give skin firmness, elasticity, and a youthful appearance. Increased levels of these proteins help counteract the gradual breakdown of collagen and the development of wrinkles and sagging that occurs with aging.

### Improve Skin Hydration

Saunas can stimulate the sebaceous glands, increasing the production of natural oils that help keep the skin hydrated and can improve its barrier function.

### Relieve Skin Conditions

The anti-inflammatory and circulation-boosting effects of sauna heat may provide symptom relief for certain inflammatory skin conditions, such as psoriasis and eczema. The heavy sweating also helps remove irritants and allergens from the skin surface. People with these conditions report reduced itching, redness, and skin irritation with regular sauna use. However, those with any skin diseases should consult their dermatologist before starting sauna therapy.

**Facilitate Inentionality**

Intentionality is a philosophical and psychological concept that refers to the mind's capacity to be about, represent, or stand for things, properties, and states of affairs. Intentions are characteristics of our mental states, but they are manifested and expressed in physical action through signals that our brain sends to various body parts, including our skin. Connections between the synapses of firing neurons form fibrous, plastic connections that hardwire our experiences into a monument of our existence.

Our skin acts as an important boundary through which our mental states interact with the world around us. It encases our bodies in a cloak of experience that allows us to sense and carry out the actions we intend to take. In a way, our skin is where the biological basis of our sense of purpose and engagement with the world meets the external environment.

**Enhance the Beauty of Bare Skin**

The skin biome is a diverse ecosystem of microorganisms that live on our skin, including bacteria, fungi, and viruses. This microbiome protects our skin from harmful pathogens, regulates our immune system, and maintains overall skin health. Regular sauna use can positively impact this delicate ecosystem through the abovementioned processes.

You can enhance the condition of the skin biome by keeping the skin clear of makeup or other skin care products, as many cosmetics and skin care products can disrupt the delicate balance of these beneficial microorganisms. Allowing this natural microbiome to thrive undisturbed helps support the skin's innate protective and regulatory functions, leading to healthier, more resilient skin in the long run.

Heat stimulation from sauna use enhances the skin's natural processes while avoiding heavy cosmetics, allowing the skin's microbiome to flourish undisturbed. This combination often leads to a clearer, more radiant complexion. The heat-induced boost in circulation and sweating and a thriving skin ecosystem support the skin's innate protective and regulatory functions. As a result, many people develop healthier, more resilient skin that appears vibrant without extensive makeup. This allows for a more natural appearance, reducing the need for cosmetic coverage while harnessing the skin-enhancing benefits of regular sauna sessions.

### My new sauna-based, bare-skin regimen

Since incorporating regular sauna sessions into my routine, I've observed a remarkable improvement in my skin's health. These positive changes have deepened my appreciation for my natural appearance, leading me to embrace a bare-skin, makeup-free look.

Sauna practice has enabled me to streamline my skincare regimen significantly. The sauna's hydrating effects have eliminated my need for moisturizer, as my skin maintains its moisture balance naturally. My long struggle with eczema came to an end with sauna practice, and I no longer need ointment. The cornerstone of my skincare routine is harnessing the rejuvenating power of "skin dunes" (refer to the image at the beginning of this chapter). These temporary skin elevations induced through dramatically increased blood flow during my daily workouts potentially enhance my skin's health and appearance. Aside from the sauna, my skincare routine is a splash of cold water on my face in the morning, washing with soap at night, and an occasional dab of Vaseline on my lips during dry conditions in conditions.

*Ending my relationship with cosmetics*

My journey with makeup began as a teenager. What started as an exciting foray into self-expression gradually became an unspoken obligation, a daily ritual influenced by advertisements promising to improve upon what I already had and beauty standards defined in the media of women in made-up faces. For five decades, cosmetics were a constant in my life, accumulating in my bathroom and becoming an integral part of my routine.

It wasn't until I downsized my living space that I was forced to confront the dilemma of what to do with the cosmetics I had accumulated but no longer used. Faced with limited storage, I had to decide what truly served me. I tossed them into the trash one Saturday night in a private ritual.

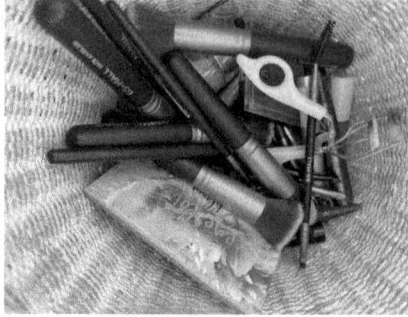

*Figure 8-2: Discarded cosmetics, brushes, and beauty tools.*

*The loveliness of liberation*

Abandoning my makeup routine has yielded multiple benefits, including time savings in my daily schedule, reduced expenses on skincare and cosmetics products, decreased exposure to potentially harmful chemicals, and a thriving natural skin balance.

This minimalist approach and newfound confidence in my appearance underscore that the sauna's benefits extend far beyond the surface level. The sauna's transformative effects work from the inside out, fostering a deep-seated comfort in my own skin.

Embracing a product-free face has become a cornerstone of my identity, not just a practical choice. This minimalist approach to skincare has led me to discover the beauty of my natural skin and reclaim my authentic self. By decluttering my cosmetics collection, I've liberated myself from a consumer culture that has long held me captive. This shift isn't merely about appearance; it's about feeling better and finding confidence in who I am fundamentally.

**Conclusion**

In conclusion, regular sauna bathing offers numerous benefits for skin health and appearance. The combination of heat exposure and induced sweating contributes to improved circulation, enhanced skin cell turnover, and deep cleansing of pores. This process aids in detoxification, removing impurities and toxins from the skin and body. Sauna use may also stimulate collagen and elastin production, promoting skin elasticity and potentially reducing signs of aging. Additionally, the practice can improve skin hydration and relieve certain inflammatory skin conditions. The skin's role as a protective barrier, temperature regulator, and sensory organ is supported and enhanced through sauna use. By promoting overall skin health, sauna bathing enhances the physical appearance and supports the skin's vital functions in maintaining overall health and well-being.

While sauna use can be an effective complementary therapy for skin conditions, it should not be used as a substitute for medical treatment. Individuals with skin conditions should consult their healthcare provider before starting any new treatment regimen, including sauna use.

# 9. Enhancing Endocrine System Functions

The endocrine system is a network of glands that produce and secrete hormones directly into the bloodstream. These hormones act as chemical messengers, traveling to target cells and organs to regulate various bodily functions, including metabolism, growth, development, reproduction, and mood.

The heat stress response from the sauna can adaptively affect the endocrine system in several ways, leading to improved hormonal regulation and stress resilience over time.

### Hypothalamic-pituitary-adrenal Axis Adaptation

As discussed in Chapter Five, the heat stress response activates the hypothalamic-pituitary-adrenal (HPA) axis, a central endocrine system component. Regular exposure to mild heat stress can make the HPA axis more efficient in responding to and recovering from stressors. This adaptation can lead to a more balanced stress response, with reduced cortisol levels and improved regulation of the HPA axis.

### Increase Growth Hormone Secretion

Growth hormone (GH) is essential for muscle growth, tissue repair, and fat metabolism. Studies have shown that sauna bathing can stimulate the release of growth hormone. Exposure to high temperatures and the subsequent cooling-down period can lead to a significant increase in

GH levels. This boost in growth hormone can promote muscle recovery, enhance fat burning, and support overall physical performance. Increased growth hormone secretion may improve body composition and overall metabolic health.

**Modulation of Sex Hormones**

Heat stress may affect the production and balance of sex hormones, such as testosterone and estrogen. These hormones are essential for reproductive health and maintaining bone density, muscle mass, and overall well-being. Sauna practice has been linked to improved reproductive health in both men and women. In men, regular sauna use has been associated with increased testosterone levels. Testosterone is essential for maintaining muscle mass, bone density, and libido. For women, sauna bathing may help to regulate menstrual cycles and alleviate symptoms of menopause, such as hot flashes and mood swings. Heat exposure can also improve circulation to the reproductive organs, promoting overall reproductive health.

**Increase Endorphin Release**

As mentioned earlier, heat stress can stimulate the release of endorphins, natural pain-relieving and mood-enhancing chemicals produced by the endocrine system. Increased endorphin levels can promote feelings of well-being and help alleviate symptoms of stress, anxiety, and depression.

**Enhance Thyroid Function**

The thyroid gland produces hormones that regulate metabolism, energy levels, and body temperature. Sauna bathing has been found to positively impact the thyroid by increasing the production and release of thyroid hormones. Thyroid hormones are crucial in regulating metabolism, energy expenditure, and thermogenesis. Improved thyroid function can contribute to better metabolic health and weight management.

**Improve Stress Resilience**

Regular exposure to mild heat stress can enhance the body's overall stress resilience by promoting adaptations in the endocrine system, leading to better coping mechanisms and reduced vulnerability to stress-related disorders.

**Improve Brown Adipose Tissue Function**

Brown adipose tissue is a type of fat that plays a role in thermogenesis, the process of producing heat. The endocrine system regulates BAT activity through various hormones and signaling pathways. Unlike white adipose tissue, which primarily stores energy, BAT is rich in mitochondria and is highly metabolically active. When activated, BAT can burn calories and generate heat, regulating body temperature and energy balance. Repeated exposure to mild heat stress may also lead to adaptive responses in the endocrine system that support BAT function. These adaptations can include increased sensitivity to hormones and enhanced production of BAT-activating factors. Improving BAT function through the heat stress response can have several potential benefits, including increased energy expenditure, improved glucose metabolism, and enhanced thermogenic capacity. BAT is discussed more thoroughly in Chapter Eleven.

**Improve Metabolic Health**

Sauna bathing can significantly impact metabolism, the process by which the body converts food and drink into energy. During a sauna session, the body's core temperature rises, causing the cardiovascular system to work harder to maintain homeostasis. Increased cardiovascular activity temporarily boosts metabolic rate, which can help the body burn more calories and fat. Sauna use and heat stress adaptively support metabolic health and flexibility through various other mechanisms. These include improved insulin sensitivity, increased glucose transporter expression, activation of AMPK (an enzyme that plays a central role in cellular energy regulation), enhanced mitochondrial function, browning of white adipose tissue, hormonal adaptations, and reduced inflammation. By promoting these adaptive responses, regular exposure to controlled heat stress can help improve glucose regulation, energy balance, and overall cellular function, thus supporting better metabolic health. Studies have shown that a single sauna session can increase metabolic rate by up to 20%, with the effects lasting for several hours after the session.

**Improve Insulin Sensitivity**

Insulin sensitivity refers to how responsive your body's cells are to the effects of insulin, a hormone produced by the pancreas. Insulin is crucial in regulating blood sugar levels by facilitating glucose uptake from the bloodstream into cells for energy or storage. When your body is more sensitive to insulin, it requires less insulin to manage blood glucose levels effectively.

Enhanced insulin sensitivity can help reduce the risk of metabolic disorders such as type 2 diabetes and metabolic syndrome. On the other hand, insulin resistance occurs when cells become less responsive to insulin, leading to higher blood sugar levels. As a result, the pancreas produces more insulin to compensate. Over time, this can lead to consistently elevated insulin levels, which may contribute to the development of type 2 diabetes and other metabolic disorders.

Regular sauna bathing has been found to improve insulin sensitivity through several mechanisms, including the activation of heat shock proteins, which will enhance the cells' response to insulin, and increased blood flow to skin and muscles, which can enhance the delivery of glucose and insulin to these tissues, improving insulin sensitivity. These mechanisms can lead to better glucose metabolism and reduced risk of metabolic disorders like type 2 diabetes and metabolic syndrome. By improving insulin sensitivity, sauna use may help maintain healthier blood sugar levels and reduce the risk of developing these conditions.

Chronic low-grade inflammation is associated with insulin resistance. Sauna use has been shown to reduce inflammation by increasing the production of anti-inflammatory cytokines and decreasing pro-inflammatory markers, thereby improving insulin sensitivity.

**Manage Weight**

Maintaining a healthy weight is essential for optimal insulin sensitivity. Sauna bathing may support weight management by increasing metabolic rate and promoting mild calorie burning. Weight management is discussed more extensively in Chapter Thirteen.

**Conclusion**

In conclusion, regular sauna bathing appears to have a significant and multi-faceted impact on the endocrine system, offering potential benefits for overall hormonal health and metabolic function. The heat stress response induced by sauna use can lead to adaptive changes in various endocrine processes, including the hypothalamic-pituitary-adrenal axis, growth hormone secretion, thyroid function, and sex hormone regulation. These adaptations can improve stress resilience, enhance metabolic health, improve insulin sensitivity, and increase brown adipose tissue function.

As research in this area continues to evolve, sauna bathing may increasingly be recognized as a valuable tool for supporting endocrine health and metabolic function as part of a comprehensive approach to wellness. While these findings are promising, the sauna use should be viewed as a complementary practice rather than a replacement for medical treatment. Individuals with pre-existing endocrine or metabolic conditions should consult with healthcare professionals before incorporating regular sauna sessions into their wellness routines.

# 10. Enhancing Immune System Functions

The immune system is the body's complex defense network against harmful pathogens and other threats. It comprises various components, including white blood cells, antibodies, and specialized organs like the thymus and spleen. The system operates through two main types of immunity: The innate immune system provides rapid, non-specific defense against pathogens, while the adaptive immune system develops targeted, long-lasting protection through specialized cells that remember and respond to specific threats. Key processes involve recognizing foreign substances, activating immune cells, neutralizing threats, and forming immunological memory. Important cells such as T cells, B cells, and macrophages play crucial roles in coordinating responses to identify, target, and destroy pathogens. The system also utilizes physical and chemical barriers like skin and stomach acid as the first lines of defense. This intricate system works continuously to maintain the body's health and fight off infections.

Exposure to heat stress through regular sauna use can bolster the immune system by activating various protective mechanisms. Sauna use further supports immune function by enhancing lymphatic function and efficiently removing waste, toxins, and pathogens from the body.

Sweating in a sauna also aids in detoxification by eliminating toxins through the skin, reducing the burden on the immune system. The heat also promotes cellular cleanup processes and may increase antibody production. Controlled heat stress acts as a form of exercise for the immune system, strengthening its response over time.

Researchers have shown that by increasing body temperature, the sauna simulates the conditions of a fever (Mace et al., 2011). The heat-induced state akin to a mild fever can enhance immune function by stimulating increased production of key immune components, including white blood cells and antibodies. White blood cells become more active, with increased production of lymphocytes and neutrophils, enhancing the body's ability to fend off pathogens. These elements strengthen the body's defenses against pathogens and illnesses, improving overall disease resistance. The warmer body environment inhibits viral and bacterial growth, potentially slowing the progression of infections (IBID). Additionally, sauna therapy reduces stress levels by promoting relaxation and the release of endorphins, which helps maintain a healthy immune system since chronic stress can weaken immune function.

**Calm Inflammation**

Inflammation is a complex biological response of the body's tissues to harmful stimuli, such as pathogens, damaged cells, or irritants. It is a protective mechanism that eliminates the cause of cell injury, clears out dead or damaged cells, and initiates tissue repair. Regular sauna sessions might help reduce chronic inflammation, which can impair immune function when persistent.

During inflammation, blood vessels undergo vasodilation, which increases blood flow to the affected area, causing the characteristic redness and warmth associated with this process. Simultaneously, the walls of these blood vessels become more permeable, allowing fluid and immune cells to move from the bloodstream into the injured tissue, resulting in swelling, or *edema*. White blood cells, particularly neutrophils and macrophages, migrate to the site of inflammation to engulf and destroy pathogens, remove debris, and release signaling molecules called cytokines that regulate the inflammatory response. Additionally, immune cells release various inflammatory mediators, such as histamine, prostaglandins, and cytokines, amplify the inflammatory response, attract more immune cells, and contribute to inflammation symptoms, including pain and fever.

While inflammation is a necessary and beneficial response to injury or infection, chronic or excessive inflammation can lead to tissue damage and contribute to the development of various diseases, such as cardiovascular disease, diabetes, and certain cancers. Sauna bathing has been shown to reduce levels of inflammatory markers such as C-reactive protein (CRP). CRP is a substance produced by the liver in response to inflammation. It is a type of acute-phase protein, meaning its levels in the blood increase when there is inflammation in the body. CRP is often measured through blood tests as a marker of inflammation and can indicate various conditions, such as infections, autoimmune diseases, cardiovascular disease, and chronic inflammatory conditions like rheumatoid arthritis and inflammatory bowel disease.

Exposure to sauna heat has been found to modulate the production of cytokines, signaling molecules that regulate inflammation and promote an overall anti-inflammatory effect. Sauna bathing may also indirectly help calm inflammation by lowering cortisol levels.

**Correct Autoimmune Disorders**

Autoimmune disorders occur when the body's immune system mistakenly attacks healthy cells, leading to chronic inflammation and various debilitating symptoms. Common autoimmune diseases include rheumatoid arthritis, lupus, multiple sclerosis, psoriasis, and Hashimoto's thyroiditis. While conventional treatments typically involve immunosuppressant drugs, lifestyle interventions like sauna therapy are showing promise as complementary approaches for managing autoimmune conditions.

One of the primary advantages is reducing inflammation by stimulating heat shock proteins (HSPs), which protect cells from stress and modulate the immune response. Sauna use also contributes to immune system modulation by shifting the balance of cytokine production towards an anti-inflammatory state and regulating immune cell activity, particularly by promoting regulatory T-cells that help control autoimmune responses.

The increased blood flow resulting from sauna sessions enhances the delivery of oxygen and nutrients to tissues, which aids in reducing inflammation and promoting healing. Regular sauna use has been shown to lower cortisol levels, a stress hormone that can exacerbate autoimmune conditions, potentially improving overall immune function. Additionally, the intense sweating induced by sauna sessions facilitates the elimination of toxins from the body, which may reduce the burden on the immune system and potentially decrease the frequency and severity of autoimmune flare-ups. These combined effects make sauna therapy a promising complementary approach for managing autoimmune disorders, though further research is needed to understand and optimize its therapeutic potential fully.

**My Immunity Response**

Since embarking on regular sauna practice, I've experienced a remarkable improvement in my ability to fight viruses and infections despite having abnormally low levels of IgG Subclass 1, one of the four types of immunoglobulin G antibodies in the immune system that help fight infections and disease (See Figure 10-1). IgG 1 antibodies are crucial for opsonization (marking pathogens for destruction) and activating the complement system, which supports other antibodies.

Like others who have compromised immunity, I previously relied heavily on antibiotics. However, antibiotics can disrupt body systems by altering the gut microbiome, affecting immune function, causing metabolic changes, contributing to antibiotic resistance, and, in some cases, increasing oxidative stress and/or impairing mitochondrial function, with these last two effects often being interconnected.

Since embarking upon my sauna practice a little more than three years ago, I haven't fallen ill once. My immunologist suggests that the sauna's heat creates a fever-like effect, probably compensating for my weakened immune system.

Cleveland Clinic MyChart
Name: Cynthia McCallister | DOB: 11/10/1960 | MRN: 90732864 | PCP: | Legal Name: Cynthia McCallister

IGG SUBCLASS 1,2,3,4
Collected on September 27, 2023 11:26 AM

Lab tests - Blood (BLOOD)

Dr. M Vera Nunez Sep 29, 10:07 PM

Result addressed on mychart message.

Results

IgG Subclass 1
Normal range: 382.4 - 928.6 mg/dL
262.8 Low
382.4 928.6

IgG Subclass 2
Normal range: 241.8 - 700.3 mg/dL
388.3
241.8 700.3

IgG Subclass 3
Normal range: 21.8 - 176.1 mg/dL
62.2
21.8 176.1

IgG Subclass 4
Normal range: 3.9 - 86.4 mg/dL
6.3
3.9 86.4

Ordering provider: Dr. M Vera Nunez
Collection date: September 27, 2023 11:26 AM
Result date: September 28, 2023 3:01 PM
Result status: Final
Resulting lab:
CLEVELAND CLINIC MAIN CAMPUS LAB
9500 Euclid Avenue
Desk L20
Cleveland OH 44195
Walter H Henricks, M.D. (Lab director)
36D0656094 (CLIA #)

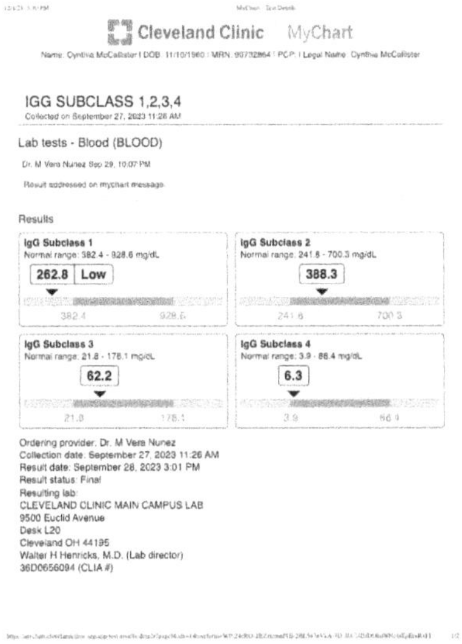

*Figure 10-1: Results from IGG Subclass 1,2,3,4 blood test*

## Conclusion

In conclusion, regular sauna use demonstrates significant potential benefits for the immune system and overall health. The heat stress induced by sauna bathing triggers a range of physiological responses that can enhance immune function, reduce chronic inflammation, and potentially aid in managing autoimmune disorders. These benefits include stimulating white blood cell production and activity, enhancing antibody production, improving lymphatic function and detoxification, reducing inflammatory markers, modulating cytokine production, and indirectly supporting immune function through stress reduction. The sauna's ability to mimic a mild fever state appears particularly beneficial in enhancing the body's natural defense mechanisms against pathogens. While these findings are promising, viewing sauna therapy as a complementary approach rather than a replacement for conventional medical treatments is crucial.

As research in this area continues to evolve, sauna bathing may increasingly be recognized as a valuable tool for supporting immune function and managing inflammatory conditions. While sauna use can be an effective complementary therapy for immune system disorders, it should not be used as a substitute for medical treatment. Individuals with immune disorders should always consult with their healthcare provider before starting any new treatment regimen, including sauna use.

# 11. ENHANCING MUSCULOSKELETAL SYSTEM FUNCTIONS

The musculoskeletal system comprises bones, muscles, tendons, ligaments, and other connective tissues that work together to provide support, stability, and movement to the body.

We usually think of the musculoskeletal system as comprising bones and muscles. The brain tells the muscles to move the bones. But muscles are not intelligent enough to carry out our intentions—akin to the gardener using a jackhammer to dig holes for daisies. The mysterious missing element of the musculoskeletal system that usually gets left out of the story is the fascia.

Fascia is a crucial connective tissue that forms a continuous network throughout the body. This web-like structure surrounds and connects various tissues and organs, including muscles, bones, nerves, and blood vessels. It serves multiple functions, providing support and structure while also helping to transmit forces and tension during movement. Fascia contains sensory receptors that contribute to proprioception, allowing us to sense our body's position and movement. It also acts as a shock absorber, aids fluid circulation, and plays a role in wound healing processes. The versatility and ubiquity of fascia make it an integral component of the body's overall function and health.

The fascia is part of the larger system known as the *myofascia*.

Myofascia is the entire integrated muscle system comprising muscle tissue (myo-) and the surrounding connective tissue (fascia). Myofascia is adaptable and responsive to stress and movement and contains sensory receptors contributing to *proprioception*. Proprioception is the body's ability to sense its position, movement, and actions without visual input. It's often referred to as our "sixth sense."

The fascia is the part of the system that envelopes muscles, organs, and other bodily structures. It acts as a continuous body-wide communication network that helps integrate sensory information and motor commands, contributing to body awareness and spatial orientation. Through its connective properties, it helps translate our intentions into action.

The musculoskeletal system executes the commands of our brain's intentions and sends information back for further coordination.

In this section, we will explore how sauna use can support the health and function of the musculoskeletal system.

**Improve Myofascial Health**

Myofascia's continuous nature throughout the body makes it significant in pain perception and management. Myofascial restrictions or trigger points often develop from injury, overuse, or postural strain, impeding mobility and causing pain. These trigger points restrict our capacity to react to the environment fully. They cause not only physical pain or discomfort, but because the impede in the successful execution of our intentions, they also can have a negative impact on mental well-being.

Understanding myofascia has led to various therapeutic approaches, such as myofascial release techniques and foam rolling, which aim to address issues like myofascial pain syndrome and improve overall physical function. Sauna therapy is a promising approach to supporting myofascial health.

The deep penetrating heat of a sauna warms the myofascial tissues, increasing extensibility and flexibility, releasing restrictions, and relieving associated muscle tension and pain.

The increased energy output required for thermoregulation in a sauna boosts metabolism and promotes better circulation in myofascial tissues. Enhanced blood flow delivers more oxygen and clears out metabolic waste products that can accumulate and cause stiffness and fatigue. The warmth and relaxation of a sauna can further reduce stress and promote a parasympathetic nervous system response, allowing the myofascial structures to let go of held tension.

### Increase Bone Strength

Recent studies have shown that regular sauna bathing can positively impact bone health and strength by improving bone density and reducing the risk of bone disease. Here's how:

#### Increased circulation

During a sauna session, the heat causes blood vessels to dilate, improving circulation throughout the body. Enhanced blood flow delivers essential nutrients and minerals to the bones, promoting their health and strength.

#### Increased vitamin D production

Exposure to heat during sauna bathing can stimulate the body's production of vitamin D. This essential vitamin plays a crucial role in calcium absorption, which is necessary for maintaining strong bones. Adequate levels of vitamin D help prevent bone loss and reduce the risk of fractures.

#### Improved stress reduction

Sauna bathing is known for its relaxing and stress-reducing effects. Chronic stress can increase cortisol levels, a hormone that can negatively impact bone health. By regularly engaging in sauna sessions, individuals can lower their stress levels and consequently reduce the detrimental effects of cortisol on bone density.

#### Improved hormone balance

Sauna bathing has been shown to positively influence hormone levels. It can help regulate hormones such as estrogen and testosterone, which play a role in maintaining bone mass. Balanced hormone levels are essential for preventing bone loss, especially in postmenopausal women who are at a higher risk of osteoporosis.

### Prevent Osteoporosis

Osteoporosis is a common bone disease that makes bones weak and more likely to break. Scientists have found that warmth might help protect bones from getting weaker, especially in mice without ovaries (which is similar to women after menopause) (Chevalier et al., 2020).

They found that their bones stayed stronger when mice were kept in a warm environment (34°C or about 93°F). The warmth helped bones keep their structure and strength in both adult female mice and young male mice. The researchers also found that the good bacteria in the gut (called the microbiome) played a role. When they took gut bacteria from mice living in warm conditions and gave it to other mice, it had similar positive effects on their bones. The warmth and the transferred gut bacteria helped reverse some bone problems caused by removing ovaries in mice. They also helped new bone to form.

The scientists discovered that warmth helps gut bacteria make more of certain helpful chemicals called polyamines. When they gave mice two specific polyamines (spermine and spermidine), it made their bones stronger. On the other hand, when they stopped the production of polyamines, the warm environment didn't help bones as much. "With heat, the synthesis of polyamines increases while their degradation is reduced. They thus affect the activity of osteoblasts (the cells that build bones) and reduce the number of osteoclasts (the cells that degrade bones). With age and menopause, the exquisite balance between the osteoclast and osteoblast activity is disrupted," explains Claire Chevalier. "However, heat, by acting on the polyamines, which we found to be partly regulated by the microbiota, can maintain the balance between these two cell groups." These findings suggest that exposure to warmth could be a prevention strategy against osteoporosis.

While sauna use can be an effective complementary therapy for bone disease, it should not be used as a substitute for medical treatment. Individuals with bone disease should always consult with their healthcare provider before starting any new treatment regimen, including sauna use.

### Improve Muscle Strength and Function

The sauna can be an invaluable tool for enhancing overall fitness and athletic performance. Integrating sauna bathing with a strength training regimen by aligning sauna use before and after weightlifting sessions accelerates muscle recovery, builds strength, and helps overcome frustrating plateaus. The strategic application of dry heat exposure complements strength training in several key ways:

***Pre-workout warm-up and activation***

The sauna's dry heat helps increase muscle temperature, heart rate, blood flow, and overall mobility—priming the body for the rigors of heavy resistance training. One study showed a 5% increase in strength with every degree.

### Post-workout recovery acceleration

Immediately after an intense lift, sauna bathing initiates a deep, cleansing sweat. It catalyzes flushing metabolic wastes like lactic acid from overtaxed muscles while increasing circulation to deliver healing nutrients. The strategic application of this "contrasting stress" compresses the normal muscle recovery timeline from days into a single restorative sauna session, allowing the same muscle groups to be trained more frequently for greater growth stimulus.

### Heat shock protein production

A key mechanism behind the sauna's recovery benefits is the production of heat shock proteins (HSPs). These protective molecules clear out damaged or misfolded proteins while fortifying healthy muscle fibers against breakdown. While strength training alone provides a potent HSP stimulus, combining it with sauna use amplifies the response of these protective proteins. More abundant HSPs mean greater reinforcement and more efficient remodeling of stronger, denser muscle fibers.

### Conclusion

In conclusion, regular sauna use significantly benefits the musculoskeletal system, supporting bone health, myofascial function, and muscle strength. The heat stress of sauna bathing triggers physiological responses that enhance overall musculoskeletal health and performance. Key benefits include increased bone strength and density, improved myofascial health, enhanced muscle strength and function, accelerated muscle recovery, and stimulated heat shock protein production. These effects are achieved through improved circulation, vitamin D production, stress reduction, hormone balance, and the direct impact of heat on tissues. While promising, sauna therapy should be viewed as a complementary approach to maintaining musculoskeletal health, not a replacement for exercise, proper nutrition, or medical treatments. As research evolves, sauna bathing may increasingly be recognized as a valuable tool for supporting musculoskeletal health, enhancing athletic performance, and potentially aiding in preventing and managing conditions like osteoporosis and myofascial pain syndrome.

While sauna use can be an effective complementary therapy for disorders of the musculoskeletal system, it should not be used as a substitute for medical treatment. Individuals with disorders of the musculoskeletal system should always consult with their healthcare provider before starting any new treatment regimen, including sauna use.

# 12. Enhancing Digestive System Functions

The digestive system breaks down food into nutrients the body can absorb and use for energy, growth, and cell repair. This process involves a series of organs and glands, including the mouth, esophagus, stomach, small intestine, large intestine, rectum, and anus, as well as accessory organs like the liver, gallbladder, and pancreas. The digestive system performs several essential functions, such as ingestion, mechanical and chemical digestion, absorption of nutrients, and elimination of waste products.

Heat stress response can improve the digestive system through several mechanisms, primarily involving physiological and molecular adaptations.

**Strengthen Intestinal Barrier Function**

The heat stress response can significantly impact gut health and function, particularly in relation to the integrity of the intestinal barrier. When the body experiences heat stress, such as during sauna use or exposure to high temperatures, it triggers a complex physiological response, including increased expression of heat shock proteins (HSPs) that play a crucial role in promoting the organization of *tight junction proteins*, special molecular structures that maintain the integrity and selective permeability of epithelial and endothelial cell barriers throughout the body, particularly in the intestinal lining.

By enhancing the expression and function of these proteins, heat stress can strengthen the intestinal barrier, reducing its permeability. This process is particularly relevant in the context of "leaky gut syndrome," also known as increased intestinal permeability, where the intestinal barrier becomes compromised, allowing the passage of potentially harmful substances from the gut lumen into the bloodstream. A more robust intestinal barrier helps prevent the movement of harmful pathogens, toxins, and undigested food particles from the gut into the systemic circulation, which could otherwise trigger immune responses and inflammation throughout the body. Furthermore, improved barrier function can contribute to overall gut health by maintaining the delicate balance of the gut microbiota, preventing dysbiosis, and supporting proper nutrient absorption.

Enhanced intestinal integrity supports local gut health and has far-reaching implications for systemic health, potentially reducing the risk of various inflammatory and autoimmune conditions associated with increased intestinal permeability.

**Improve Gut Microbiota Composition**

The gut microbiota, also known as gut flora or gut microbiome, refers to the vast community of microorganisms that reside in the human gastrointestinal tract, primarily in the large intestine. This complex ecosystem consists of trillions of microorganisms, including bacteria, fungi, viruses, and other microbes, with bacteria being the most abundant and well-studied. The gut microbiota plays a crucial role in human health, influencing various aspects of physiology, including digestion, nutrient absorption, protection against pathogenic microorganisms, promoting the growth of beneficial bacteria, and inhibiting harmful ones metabolism, immune function, and even brain health. It helps break down food components that human cells cannot digest, produces essential vitamins and short-chain fatty acids, protects against pathogens, and interacts with the immune system. A healthy gut microbiome supports all body systems. Maintaining a diverse and balanced gut microbiota is increasingly recognized as important for overall health and well-being.

The gut microbiota composition is unique to each individual and can be influenced by factors such as diet, lifestyle, genetics, medication use, and environmental exposures. It can also be influenced by heat stress. Increased core body temperature creates an environment that may promote the growth of beneficial bacteria while inhibiting some harmful ones. Heat exposure induces the production of heat shock proteins, which can enhance gut barrier function and support a healthier microbiome. Improved blood flow to the gut due to heat exposure can enhance nutrient delivery to beneficial bacteria and aid in waste removal. Heat-induced stress reduction is associated with a more diverse and balanced microbiome. Sweating may help eliminate toxins that could negatively impact gut bacteria. Heat exposure can also influence metabolism, potentially creating conditions that favor beneficial bacteria and modulate immune function, which closely interacts with the gut microbiome.

### Improve Nutrient Delivery

During heat stress, blood flow to the gut can increase to dissipate heat and supply necessary nutrients and oxygen to the tissues. This improved circulation allows nutrients to be more effectively delivered to cells and tissues, supporting their growth, repair, and overall health.

Also, because sweating during sauna sessions can help the body eliminate toxins and waste products that may interfere with nutrient absorption and utilization, sauna bathing can create a more favorable environment for the body to use the nutrients it receives from food and supplements.

### Improve Stress-related Digestive Dysregulation

Sauna bathing offers a powerful approach to improving stress-related digestive dysregulation through multiple physiological mechanisms. When the body experiences chronic stress, it maintains a persistent "fight or flight" response, diverting blood flow away from the digestive system. Over time, this can lead to a cascade of digestive issues, including bloating, constipation, and gut lining inflammation. Sauna sessions counteract this stress response by inducing deep relaxation and redirecting blood flow back to the digestive organs. This improved circulation enhances digestive function and reduces the risk of gastrointestinal problems.

Additionally, the heat stress response during sauna use influences the release of stress hormones, particularly cortisol. Cortisol plays a crucial role in gut health by improving the coordinated contractions of intestinal muscles and enhancing gut motility. It also stimulates the secretion of digestive fluids and enzymes, essential for breaking down food and aiding nutrient absorption. Regular sauna use helps maintain a balanced digestive process by promoting proper regulation of these stress hormones. This hormonal equilibrium is key in preventing stress-related digestive disorders, such as irritable bowel syndrome (IBS). Through its combined effects on blood flow, stress hormone modulation, and digestive secretions, sauna bathing presents a holistic method for addressing stress-induced digestive dysregulation and promoting overall gastrointestinal health.

**Stimulate Peristalsis**

The increased body temperature during a sauna session can stimulate peristalsis, the rhythmic contractions of the digestive tract that help move food through the system, relieve constipation, and promote regular bowel movements.

**Conclusion**

In conclusion, regular sauna use significantly benefits the digestive system through various physiological and molecular mechanisms. These include enhanced production of heat shock proteins, strengthened intestinal barrier function, improved gut microbiota composition, reduced inflammation, enhanced cellular repair, improved blood flow and nutrient delivery, better stress hormone modulation, improved digestion through relaxation, stimulated peristalsis, and support for natural detoxification processes. Collectively, these effects contribute to a healthier, more efficient digestive system, which in turn supports overall well-being due to the crucial role of digestion in nutrient absorption, immune function, and even mood regulation.

While promising, sauna therapy should be viewed as a complementary approach to maintaining digestive health alongside a balanced diet and regular exercise. While sauna use can be an effective complementary therapy for digestive conditions, it should not be used as a substitute for medical treatment. Individuals with digestive conditions should consult their healthcare provider before starting any new treatment regimen, including sauna use.

# 13. ENHANCING SYSTEMIC FUNCTIONS

Regular sauna practice has been found to provide a wide range of positive effects on all of the body's systems and to have an overall positive effect on aspects of systemic body functioning. This chapter will explore how sauna use can benefit the body's holistic functioning.

**Reduce Mortality Risk**

Regular sauna bathing is associated with a lower mortality risk. A growing body of research has explored the potential mechanisms behind these benefits, shedding light on how sauna use might contribute to a longer, healthier life. As discussed in previous chapters, one of the primary ways sauna bathing may reduce mortality risk is through its positive effects on cardiovascular health and how it can help lower blood pressure, improve endothelial function, and promote better overall cardiovascular function. Additionally, the relaxation and stress-reducing properties of sauna bathing can profoundly impact mental well-being. Given the strong link between chronic stress and various health problems, including an increased risk of mortality, the ability of saunas to promote relaxation and alleviate stress may play a significant role in their potential life-extending benefits.

Beyond its cardiovascular and stress-reducing effects, sauna exposure has been shown to improve respiratory function, particularly in individuals with conditions such as asthma and chronic obstructive pulmonary disease (COPD). Sweat induced by sauna use may also help eliminate toxins from the body, potentially lowering the risk of certain diseases. Additionally, regular sauna bathing has been found to stimulate the immune system, enhance insulin sensitivity, and provide relief from chronic pain conditions.

Several studies have investigated the relationship between sauna use and reduced mortality risk due to reduced cardiovascular disease, reduced hypertension, and lower levels of inflammation and oxidative stress. Here are summaries of these notable studies:

• Laukkanen et al. (2015) followed 2,315 middle-aged men from Eastern Finland for a median of 20.7 years, finding that increased frequency and duration of sauna bathing were inversely associated with the risk of sudden cardiac death, fatal coronary heart disease, fatal cardiovascular disease, and all-cause mortality.

• Laukkanen et al. (2018) followed 1,688 men and women aged 53-74 for a median of 15 years and found that regular sauna bathing (4-7 times per week) was associated with a significantly reduced risk of fatal cardiovascular disease events and all-cause mortality compared to those who had one sauna session per week.

• Zaccardi et al. (2017) followed 1,621 middle-aged men without hypertension at baseline for a median of 24.7 years. The results showed that frequent sauna bathing (4-7 sessions per week) was associated with a reduced risk of hypertension compared to those who had one sauna session per week.

• Kunutsor et al. (2018) followed 2,269 men aged 42-61 for a median of 24.7 years and found that frequent sauna bathing (4-7 sessions per week) was associated with lower levels of inflammation and oxidative stress, which may contribute to the reduced risk of mortality observed in other studies.

These studies suggest that regular sauna use, particularly 4-7 sessions per week, may be associated with a reduced risk of cardiovascular disease and all-cause mortality. However, more research is needed to establish a causal relationship and to determine the optimal frequency and duration of sauna sessions for health benefits.

### Slow Aging

Usually, when we think of a person's age, we refer to their chronological age, the number of years a person has been alive. However, aging can also be understood in biological terms. A person's biological age refers to the physiological state of their cells, tissues, and organs relative to their chronological age. Various factors, such as genetics, lifestyle, environment, and disease history, influence the rate of biological aging. Depending on these factors, two people of the same chronological age may have different biological ages. For example, a person who maintains a healthy lifestyle, including a balanced diet, regular exercise, and stress management, may have a lower biological age compared to someone of the same chronological age who engages in unhealthy behaviors like smoking, excessive alcohol consumption, and a sedentary lifestyle.

Humans evolved to live a relatively long time—into the sixth and seventh decade—compared to chimpanzees, who live only until age 15 (Gurven & Kaplan, 2007). Research suggests that the extended human lifespan evolved as an adaptation to a diet rich in animal proteins. Natural selection favored longevity because hunting skills, crucial for obtaining these nutrient-dense foods, tend to peak after age 40 (Kaplan et al. 2000 & 2007). This evolutionary pressure allowed humans to benefit from the accumulated hunting experience of older individuals, contributing to the group's survival and leading to our comparatively long lifespans.

While humans have the biological capacity to live a relatively long time, an individual's lifespan is influenced by the aging process, which encompasses a variety of biological, genetic, and environmental factors. At the cellular level, aging involves accumulating damage from oxidative stress, DNA mutations, and protein misfolding, which impair cellular function and lead to age-related diseases. If not repaired properly, this damage can lead to mutations and epigenetic changes that disrupt normal cellular function. Reduction in the function and number of stem cells decreases as we age. Stem cells are responsible for replenishing damaged or lost tissue cells. Genetic factors also play a significant role, with certain genes promoting longevity while others may predispose individuals to diseases that shorten lifespan. Mitochondria, the cell's powerhouses, become less efficient with age, leading to increased oxidative stress, reduced energy production, and impaired cellular function. One of the key aspects of cellular aging is telomere shortening; as cells divide, these protective caps at the ends of chromosomes gradually wear down, eventually leading to cellular senescence or death when they become too short.

Additionally, the accumulation of *senescent* cells increases with age. Senescent cells are cells that have stopped dividing but remain metabolically active. They can release harmful substances that promote chronic inflammation and aging.

Beyond cellular changes, aging is marked by metabolic and hormonal shifts, such as decreased insulin sensitivity and altered levels of growth and sex hormones, all of which impact health and longevity. The immune system also declines with age in a process known as *immunosenescence*, the age-related decline in immune system function. Immunosenescence is characterized by reduced production and diversity of immune cells, chronic inflammation, and impaired immune responses, leading to increased susceptibility to infections, cancer, and autoimmune diseases in older individuals.

Lifestyle and environmental factors, such as diet, exercise, and exposure to toxins, further influence the aging process, with healthier habits mitigating some detrimental effects. Social and psychological factors, including strong social connections and good mental health, are also crucial for healthy aging and increased lifespan, highlighting the complex interplay of multiple factors in determining longevity.

Heat stress and sauna use positively influence the deceleration of the rate of aging by activating several biological mechanisms that counteract age-related decline. One of the key benefits is the induction of heat shock proteins (HSPs), which help stabilize and refold damaged proteins, thereby mitigating the harmful effects of oxidative stress and protein misfolding, contributing to maintaining cellular function and reducing the progression of age-related diseases. Additionally, regular sauna sessions improve mitochondrial function, enhancing cellular energy production and reducing oxidative stress. Improved mitochondrial efficiency can slow aging and lower metabolic disease risk. Furthermore, some studies suggest that heat stress may help maintain telomere length, delaying cellular senescence and promoting longevity. Heat stress also stimulates stem cell activation, enhancing tissue repair and regeneration, which counteracts the decline in stem cell function and number associated with aging.

Sauna use also impacts metabolic and hormonal health, improving insulin sensitivity and promoting the release of growth hormones, which can counteract some metabolic and hormonal shifts that accompany aging. Moreover, heat stress boosts the immune system, counteracting immunosenescence and making the body more resilient to infections, cancer, and other age-related diseases. Sauna use reduces chronic inflammation by lowering pro-inflammatory cytokine levels, which is crucial as chronic inflammation significantly contributes to aging and many age-related diseases. By reducing inflammation, saunas promote healthier aging. Regular sauna use can positively influence the aging process, enhancing cellular repair mechanisms, optimizing metabolic and hormonal functions, boosting immune health, and reducing inflammation, all of which contribute to increased longevity and a healthier lifespan.

### Manage Weight

While sauna use should not be considered a standalone solution for weight loss, it can be a valuable complement to a comprehensive weight management program. The heat stress induced by sauna sessions can support weight management through several mechanisms, discussed in previous chapters:

#### Increased metabolic rate

Exposure to high temperatures during sauna use can temporarily increase the body's metabolic rate. As the body works to maintain its core temperature, it expends energy, increasing calorie burn. While the number of calories burned during a sauna session may be modest, regular sauna use can have a cumulative effect over time.

#### Improved insulin sensitivity

Heat stress has been shown to improve insulin sensitivity, which is essential for maintaining a healthy weight. Improved insulin sensitivity helps the body more effectively regulate blood sugar levels, reducing the likelihood of excess glucose being stored as fat.

### Hormone regulation

Sauna use can influence the production and release of hormones that play a role in appetite control and fat storage. For example, heat stress can increase the production of growth hormone, which helps to build and maintain lean muscle mass, and can also stimulate the release of norepinephrine, which promotes fat breakdown.

### Stress reduction

Chronic stress is often associated with weight gain, as it can lead to overeating and the production of cortisol, a hormone that promotes fat storage. Regular sauna use can help reduce stress levels, promote relaxation, and potentially reduce stress-related eating behaviors.

### Improved sleep quality

Adequate, high-quality sleep is crucial for maintaining a healthy weight. Sauna use can promote better sleep by reducing stress, relaxing muscles, and inducing a sense of calm. Improved sleep can help regulate appetite hormones and reduce cravings for high-calorie foods.

### Enhanced exercise recovery

For those engaging in regular exercise as part of their weight management program, sauna use can aid post-exercise recovery. Heat stress can help to relax muscles, reduce inflammation, and improve circulation, allowing individuals to recover more quickly and maintain a consistent exercise routine.

While sauna use can be an effective complementary therapy for weight management, it should not be used as a substitute for medical treatment. Individuals with weight problems should always consult with their healthcare provider before starting any new treatment regimen, including sauna use.

### Relieve Chronic Pain

Chronic pain is a debilitating condition that affects millions of people worldwide. It can stem from various causes, such as injuries, arthritis, fibromyalgia, illnesses, or even emotional stress. While there are numerous treatment options available, including medication and physical therapy, many individuals are turning to alternative methods for relief. One such method that has gained popularity in recent years is the use of saunas.

The therapeutic effects of sauna on chronic pain can be attributed to several factors:

### Improved muscle relaxation

The heat generated by a sauna can help relax tense muscles and reduce joint stiffness. These benefits can be particularly beneficial for individuals with conditions such as arthritis or fibromyalgia, where muscle tension and joint stiffness are common symptoms.

### Improved circulation

The increased blood circulation during a sauna session can help deliver oxygen and nutrients to the muscles and joints, promoting healing and reducing inflammation. This increased blood flow can also help flush out toxins and metabolic waste products that contribute to pain and discomfort.

### Improved stress reduction

The relaxation response during a sauna session can help reduce stress and promote well-being. Chronic pain is often associated with high levels of stress and anxiety, which can exacerbate symptoms and make it difficult to cope with daily activities. By promoting relaxation and reducing stress, sauna use can help to break this cycle and improve overall quality of life.

### Reduced inflammation

Heat shock proteins (HSPs) induced by heat stress in the sauna help alleviate pain by protecting cells from damage and reducing inflammation. Additionally, heat stress can reduce the levels of pro-inflammatory cytokines, further contributing to the decrease in inflammation-associated pain.

### Decreased pain perception

The activation of Heat Shock Factor 1 (HSF1) is another key mechanism through which sauna use can alleviate chronic pain. HSF1 is a transcription factor that translocates to the nucleus and promotes gene expression, protecting cells from stress and reducing inflammation. Heat stress can modulate the activity of pain receptors, leading to a temporary increase in pain threshold and a reduction in the sensation of chronic pain.

### Increased endorphin release

Sauna use can also enhance the release of endogenous opioids, such as endorphins and enkephalins, which bind to opioid receptors in the nervous system, effectively reducing pain perception. Furthermore, the heat shock proteins produced during sauna sessions help to mitigate oxidative stress by maintaining cellular homeostasis and preventing the accumulation of damaged proteins and reactive oxygen species (ROS). This process, in turn, can help reduce pain associated with oxidative damage.

### *Neuroprotection*

Heat stress provides neuroprotection by preventing neuronal apoptosis (cell death) and promoting the survival of neurons under stress conditions. This process helps preserve the nervous system's integrity and reduce pain signals. Additionally, sauna use can improve mitochondrial function and cellular energy production, leading to better mitochondrial health, reduced cellular stress, and decreased inflammation, all contributing to alleviating chronic pain.

Through the combination of these various mechanisms, the heat stress response induced by the sauna offers a powerful means of addressing chronic pain through its anti-inflammatory, neuroprotective, and analgesic effects.

Relief from chronic pain can lead to a better quality of life and a more balanced body. While sauna use can be an effective complementary therapy for chronic pain, it should not be used as a substitute for medical treatment. Individuals with chronic pain should always consult with their healthcare provider before starting any new treatment regimen, including sauna use.

### Conclusion

In conclusion, this chapter has explored the profound and wide-ranging benefits of regular sauna practice on holistic body functioning. From reducing mortality risk to slowing aging, managing weight, and alleviating chronic pain, sauna use offers a multifaceted approach to enhancing overall health and longevity.

As research in this field continues to evolve, it becomes increasingly clear that regular sauna use can be a valuable addition to a healthy lifestyle. However, it's crucial to remember that sauna practice should complement, not replace, medical treatments, and individuals should consult healthcare providers before incorporating sauna use into their health regimens, especially those with pre-existing conditions.

Ultimately, the ancient practice of sauna bathing, supported by modern scientific understanding, offers a promising, non-pharmacological approach to enhancing systemic body functioning and promoting longevity. As we continue to uncover the full potential of heat stress therapies, sauna use stands out as a holistic method for optimizing health and well-being in our increasingly long-lived society.

# PART THREE

## SAUNA PRACTICE

*We are what we repeatedly do.*

— ARISTOTLE

Embarking on a regular sauna routine isn't just about adding a new habit to your lifestyle—it's a journey of physical, mental, and spiritual transformation. This transformative journey will inspire, motivate, and ultimately lead you to a healthier, more resilient version of yourself.

In the following chapters, you will discover the knowledge and tools to craft a personalized sauna routine that aligns with your unique goals and preferences. From beginner protocols to advanced techniques for optimizing your body's performance, this section is your guide to making sauna bathing an integral part of your self-care regimen.

# 14. Establishing a Sauna Routine

While the latent physiological capacities of thermoregulation described in Chapter Two lie within all of us, their effective function requires training through continual, ongoing exposure to intense heat. In other words, while all humans have the potential physiological capacity to withstand long periods of exposure to extreme heat, they only come into existence when used.

Modern technologies enable many of us to live in bubbles of comfort at about 70° Fahrenheit all year without stimulating our innate thermoregulatory capacities. Our comfort mindsets urge us to avoid temperature extremes—to cool ourselves with summertime air conditioning and crank up the heat in wintertime. In a way, modern humans have crippled themselves with comfort.

We live in an era in which our comforts compromise our health. In the long term, protection from temperature extremes robs us of opportunities to use thermoregulatory capacities that strengthen the body and prevent disease. Just as we need to make a deliberate effort to exercise or eat a whole-food diet, we need to become intentional about training our bodies to efficiently regulate temperature extremes by using our thermoregulatory capacities.

If you are like most people, you haven't trained your body to tolerate extended exposure to intense heat. In intense heat, you might experience the stress response that turns on your body's flight reaction. However, you can strengthen your thermoregulatory capacities through disciplined and intentional exposure to increasing amounts of heat. As you embark upon a journey into sauna practice, you will take affirmative steps to train your body to use its thermoregulatory capacities to maintain health and well-being efficiently.

This chapter is intended to introduce you to the basics of sauna practice. The chapter will help you prepare for what to expect as you begin your sauna practice routine and provide guidance in helping you establish a system for training your body to tolerate increasing levels or doses of heat over time.

By the end of this chapter, you will have a deeper understanding of the routines and practices that can make the sauna experience rewarding. Whether you are a seasoned sauna-goer or a curious newcomer, establishing your routines will fully allow you to reap the transformative power of the ancient sauna tradition.

**Sauna Access**

To find access to a sauna, start by exploring local gyms and fitness centers, which often include saunas in their facilities. Check nearby day spas, wellness centers, and community recreation facilities, as these may offer sauna sessions as standalone services or as part of broader packages. Some apartment complexes and university recreation centers also provide saunas for residents or students. When searching, consider factors like cleanliness, privacy, and operating hours to find the best fit for your sauna practice.

If commercial options are limited in your area, consider joining or starting a sauna co-op, where a group shares a private sauna (See Appendix B). As the benefits of regular sauna use are becoming increasingly recognized, waiting for governments or communities to provide public sauna facilities in areas where other options don't exist may mean missing out on crucial health and wellness opportunities. Consider initiating a community project to bring a public sauna to your area. See Appendix C: Organizing a Community Sauna Wellness Initiative.

**Sauna Culture**

Navigating the cultural space of the sauna is a crucial aspect of sauna practice. Saunas aren't merely hot rooms for relaxation and health benefits; they are shared spaces where etiquette, respect, and mindfulness significantly create a harmonious and enjoyable experience for all users. Understanding the unwritten rules and customs of sauna behavior is essential to ensure that everyone can fully immerse themselves in the sauna's comforting atmosphere without causing discomfort or offense to others. Sauna culture can vary significantly across different settings, each with its unique atmosphere, customs, and expectations. The experience of using a sauna in a gym, community center, or spa can differ in terms of etiquette, social dynamics, and the overall purpose of the sauna session. Learning to navigate the space properly can make your sauna practice more satisfying.

### Gym saunas

In a gym setting, saunas are often viewed as a post-workout amenity focused on physical recovery and relaxation. Users are typically there to unwind after a strenuous exercise, relieve muscle tension, and promote cardiovascular health. Gym saunas may have a more utilitarian atmosphere, with less emphasis on social interaction and more on individual recovery. Conversations tend to be limited. Users often wear workout attire.

### Community center saunas

Community center saunas often serve as a gathering place for members to socialize, relax, and connect. Etiquette in a community center sauna may emphasize respect, consideration, and maintaining a friendly environment. As the sauna becomes a hub for community bonding and connection, users are more likely to engage in conversations and build a sense of camaraderie.

### Spa saunas

In a spa setting, saunas are typically part of a holistic wellness experience, focusing on relaxation, rejuvenation, and stress relief. Spa saunas often have a more luxurious and tranquil ambiance. Etiquette in a spa sauna may be more formal and centered around creating a peaceful and meditative environment. Users are encouraged to maintain a quiet atmosphere, avoid engaging in loud conversations, and respect others' space and privacy. Spa saunas may also have designated silent areas or times to promote deep relaxation and introspection.

**Sauna Etiquette**

Despite differences in the purpose of various sauna types, some universal aspects of sauna culture apply across all settings. These include maintaining cleanliness, practicing good hygiene, being mindful of others' comfort, and respecting the sauna space and equipment. Regardless of the setting, the ultimate goal of sauna use remains the same: to promote physical, mental, and emotional well-being through the power of heat, relaxation, and communal experience. Here are some tips to help you observe sauna etiquette:

- Cleanliness: Always sit or lie on a clean towel to maintain hygiene and prevent the spread of bacteria. Bring an additional towel or washcloth to wipe off excess sweat.
- Clothing: In most public saunas, wearing a swimsuit or wrapping yourself in a towel is customary. Nudity may be acceptable in private or gender-specific saunas, but always check the facility's guidelines.
- Noise: Maintain a quiet and peaceful atmosphere in the sauna. Avoid loud conversations, phone calls, or other disruptive behavior that may disturb other users.
- Scents: Avoid using strong perfumes, colognes, or essential oils in the sauna, as they can be overwhelming in a heated environment and may cause discomfort to others.
- Space: Be mindful of personal space and avoid overcrowding. If the sauna is full, wait for a spot to become available before entering, or plan to sit on the floor or stand by a wall. You can lie down if there's room. Try lying on your back with feet on the ground, hip width's distance apart, providing reclining comfort in minimal space. Never lie down when it is evident that other users need space to sit.
- Electronics: Keep electronic devices, such as phones and tablets, outside the sauna to prevent damage and maintain a relaxing environment.

- Doors: Close the sauna door gently to minimize heat loss and avoid disturbing others.
- Culture and customs: Sauna customs may vary depending on the country or culture. Always observe any specific rules or guidelines posted at the sauna facility.

### Establishing a Sauna Practice Routine

Creating a consistent sauna routine can help you maximize your sessions' health benefits and enjoyment. Here are some tips to help you establish a sauna routine that works for you:

#### Identify your objective

Determine your primary goal for using the sauna. Are you looking to relax and unwind, socialize with friends or family, cleanse and heal your body, or improve your cardiovascular health by increasing your maximum cardiac output? Understanding your objective will help you tailor your routine accordingly.

#### Determine session frequency

Decide how often you want to use the sauna. Two to three sessions per week can provide significant benefits, but greater frequency can achieve more robust results. Daily sauna bathing results in dramatic results, which diminish with fewer days of exposure. Adjust the frequency of your practice based on your objectives, preferences, and health status.

#### Set a regular schedule

Choose a time that fits your daily routine, whether in the morning, after work, or before bedtime. Try to maintain this schedule consistently to make it a habit.

#### Manage session durations

If you're new to the sauna, your body might only tolerate shorter sessions of 10-15 minutes. You can gradually increase the duration as you adapt to heat and increase tolerance. You can stack several short intervals within a more extended session if you take breaks between intervals to cool down adequately and lower your heart rate. A cold shower will allow you to cool more quickly than sitting out to cool at room temperature.

#### Manage heat exposure

Ideally, start with a lower temperature (around 150°F/65°C) and gradually increase it to your comfort level. However, the temperature in saunas housed in larger facilities, like gyms or clubs, is typically between 160-200°F. In these situations, you can still adjust the temperature to which your body is exposed by *working the shelves* to regulate your temperature and heart rate. Sit on the highest shelf for greater heat intensity to raise your heart rate, or sit on the lower bench (or the floor) for a more moderate temperature to slow your heart rate.

The temperature differences between shelves can vary, but generally, there is about a 20-30°F (11-17°C) difference between each level. For example, if the bottom bench is around 130°F (54°C) and closer to the floor, where the cooler air settles. The middle bench might be about 160°F (71°C). This level provides a good balance of heat and comfort for many sauna users. The top bench could reach 190°F (88°C) or above. The hot air rises to the top, making this level the most intense heat experience.

### *Monitor and intentionally modulate your heart rate*

Your cardiovascular fitness level, heart rate, and training objectives should determine each exposure or interval's length and temperature intensity. If you are a beginner or have poor cardiovascular health, start conservatively with a level of exposure that enables you to achieve a low to moderate level of intensity. If you suffer from a medical condition, get approval from your healthcare provider before beginning sauna practice. If your fitness level is intermediate or advanced, you can start with a level of exposure that enables you to achieve a moderate to high-intensity workout. The next chapter will present everything you need to know to find your fitness level and target heart rate.

Sitting up and lying down can be an effective strategy to moderate heart rate while in a sauna. When you're in a sauna, your body temperature rises, causing blood vessels to dilate and increasing blood flow to the skin to help cool the body. This increased blood flow puts extra demand on the cardiovascular system, leading to an increase in heart rate. When sitting up or standing in a sauna, gravity pulls blood down into the lower extremities, which can reduce blood flow back to the heart (venous return), causing a further increase in heart rate as the heart works harder to maintain adequate circulation. However, when you lie down in a sauna, you minimize the effect of gravity on blood circulation, allowing blood to more easily return to the heart, increasing venous return, and reducing the workload on the heart, which may result in a decrease in heart rate compared to sitting up or standing. By alternating between sitting up and lying down, you can help regulate your heart rate, with sitting up allowing your heart rate to increase, providing a gentle form of cardiovascular exercise, and lying down giving your heart a chance to recover and reducing the overall strain on your cardiovascular system.

### Hydrate

Drink plenty of water before, during, and after your sauna session to stay hydrated. It is necessary to

keep hydrated during prolonged sauna sessions. I drink two liters of water throughout a 90-minute sauna session.

Drink from m*etal insulated bottles*, such as those made from stainless steel, are an excellent choice for the sauna. These bottles feature double-wall insulation that helps maintain the temperature of your water, keeping it cool even in the hot sauna environment. Alternatively, opt for a heat-resistant plastic bottle designed for high-temperature situations. These bottles are made from Tritan or BPA-free plastics that can withstand the sauna's heat without leaching chemicals into your water. Wash your bottle after each use, or uncap it and let it air dry for several minutes to kill microbes before using it again.

### Bathe on an empty stomach

Avoiding a heavy meal before a sauna session is advisable because it helps prevent various discomforts and potential health risks. After a heavy meal, blood flow is directed towards the digestive system, but a sauna requires increased blood flow to the skin for cooling, leading to conflicting demands that can cause discomfort or fainting. The sauna's heat can also slow digestion, resulting in bloating, nausea, or general discomfort. There is also a heightened risk of dehydration, as both digestion and sweating require water. Furthermore, an increased heart rate from eating a heavy meal and the sauna's heat can strain the cardiovascular system, particularly in individuals with heart conditions. Therefore, eating light meals and staying hydrated before using a sauna is recommended.

### *Avoid alcohol*

Avoiding alcohol before a sauna session is crucial due to several health and safety reasons. Alcohol is a diuretic, which increases urine production and can lead to dehydration. Combining this with the heavy sweating in a sauna significantly raises the risk of dehydration. Additionally, alcohol impairs the body's ability to regulate temperature and its perception of heat, which can prevent you from realizing when you're becoming overheated, increasing the risk of heat exhaustion or heat stroke. Alcohol also affects judgment, coordination, and balance, making it more likely to experience accidents or injuries in the sauna. Furthermore, both alcohol consumption and the heat of a sauna cause vasodilation, or the widening of blood vessels, which can lead to a dangerous drop in blood pressure, causing dizziness or fainting. For these reasons, it is highly recommended to avoid alcohol before using a sauna to ensure safety and well-being.

### *Create an optimal environment*

Enhance your sauna experience by playing soothing music, practicing meditation or deep breathing exercises, or connecting with others socially. A prolonged sauna session might include a little of each.

### *Cool down properly*

After your sauna session, let your body cool down gradually. Take a warm shower, followed by a cooler one, and rest for at least 10 minutes before resuming your daily activities. After a 90-minute sauna practice, I continue sweating for about an hour.

### *Listen to your body*

Pay attention to how you feel during and after your sauna sessions. If you experience discomfort or feel unwell, adjust your routine or consult a healthcare professional.

### *Be consistent*

Consistency is key when establishing a sauna routine. By making sauna sessions a regular part of your self-care regimen and aligning them with your objectives, you'll be better positioned to reap their numerous health benefits.

### **Embrace the Principle of Hormesis**

The Latin phrase "per aspera ad astra" means "through hardships to the stars." It emphasizes the idea that perseverance through adversity makes us stronger.

This concept relates closely to the principle of *hormesis*. In the phenomenon of hormesis, a low dose of a potentially harmful agent (like heat or toxins) benefits an organism. In contrast, a higher dose of the same agent can be detrimental. This concept is often summarized by saying, "What doesn't kill you makes you stronger."

The mechanisms underlying hormesis aren't fully understood but may involve activating cellular stress response pathways, such as heat shock proteins and DNA repair mechanisms, which can help protect against future insults and promote overall health and longevity.

Strive to structure your sauna practice so that, with each session, you are stimulating the hormetic response. The exposure should be strong enough to have a beneficial effect, such as raising your heart rate, but not so much as detrimental. Heat stress can benefit overall functioning, but excessive heat exposure can lead to damage and dysfunction. In the next chapter, I'll explain how you can develop a training protocol that supports a long-term adaptive hormetic response.

### Sauna Tips and Trappings

Explore different ways to enhance the sauna experience. Here are some to consider:

#### Feet up the wall

"Feet up the wall" is a simple and restorative yoga pose called Viparita Karani. It involves lying on your back with your legs extended vertically up a wall. Feet up the wall is said to reduce stress and promote relaxation, improve circulation, relieve tired or swollen feet, help relieve mild backache and headaches, calm the mind, and aid in sleep. The combination of heat from the sauna and the inverted position of the elevation of the feet can cause a sudden increase in blood flow to your feet and toes. This rush of blood may cause a tingling or stinging sensation, particularly if you're not used to it. The pose is generally safe for most people, but those with certain eye conditions, such as glaucoma or neck injuries, should consult a healthcare professional before practicing it.

#### Sauna cap

A sauna hat, typically made of wool or felt, is a conical or cylindrical cap that covers the head and ears during sauna sessions. Wearing a sauna hat offers several benefits that enhance the overall sauna experience:

- Heat Protection: The hat shields the head, face, and ears from the sauna's intense heat, reducing the risk of overheating and discomfort.
- Even Heat Distribution: By preventing excessive heat from reaching the head, a sensitive area for temperature regulation, the hat helps distribute heat evenly throughout the body.
- Hair Protection: High temperatures can damage hair, causing it to become dry and brittle. A sauna hat traps moisture, preventing the hair from drying out due to the heat.
- Hygiene: The hat absorbs moisture from the scalp, keeping sweat from dripping onto the face and maintaining cleanliness.
- Comfort: Wearing a sauna hat prevents the uncomfortable sensation of direct, intense heat on the scalp, allowing users to stay longer.
- Tradition: In some cultures, particularly in Finland, where saunas originated, wearing a sauna hat is a long-standing tradition and proper etiquette.

### Plastic sand timer

Digital and electronic tools for heart rate monitoring, like cell phones and wearable heart rate monitors, aren't designed to withstand the sauna's high temperatures. To monitor your heart rate in the sauna's heat, use a plastic 15- or 30-second sand timer. Using a 15-second timer, take your pulse and multiply by four to get your heart rate. Using a 30-second timer, take your pulse and multiply by two.

### Microfiber towel

Always sit on a towel in the sauna. Microfiber towels are ideal for saunas because they are hygienic, highly absorbent, quick-drying, compact, and durable.

### Cotton tea towel

Bring a small, lightweight towel into the sauna to dry facial sweat. Consider using a 100% ringspun cotton tea towel. The light cotton towel dries quickly and can be used throughout the sauna session.

### Electrolyte supplements

Certain electrolytes, such as magnesium, potassium, calcium, sodium, and chloride, are lost through sweat. To avoid cramping and other symptoms of dehydration, consider electrolyte supplementation. You can keep a liquid supplement in your sauna bag and add a few drops to your water bottle before your session or take supplements in pill or capsule form. I have found adequate calcium, sodium, and chloride levels through my diet, but I need to supplement with potassium and magnesium occasionally.

### Record Your Journey

To deepen your connection with your sauna journey, consider journaling your experiences. Note any changes in your physical, mental, and emotional well-being, and observe how your perspective on health and life evolves. By sharing these stories with the sauna community, you contribute to a collective narrative of healing and transformation.

### Practice Presence

To get the most out of the sauna experience, it is essential to approach your sauna practice with the right mindset. While it may be tempting to view the sauna as a place to catch up on work or scroll through your phone, doing so can prevent you from fully embracing the stillness of the sauna environment for introspection and the communal benefits that sauna culture offers. Instead, by practicing presence and savoring the stillness of the sauna space or engaging in authentic conversations and building relationships, you can tap into the fullest benefits of sauna practice.

### Conclusion

As you establish habits and routines of sauna practice, know that you are gradually training your body to tolerate increasing heat levels and transforming into a stronger, more empowered version of yourself.

# Unlock the Power of Wellness: Your Review Matters!

"Small acts, when multiplied by millions of people, can transform the world." - Howard Zinn

You've learned about the transformative benefits of the sauna. Now, you can help others discover this path to better health and well-being by leaving a review. Your review can:

1. Guide those seeking positive change in their lives
2. Help make sauna benefits accessible to everyone
3. Spread awareness about this powerful wellness tool

**Why Your Voice Matters:**

- People trust authentic experiences
- Your insights can inspire others to take the first step
- Each review brings us closer to a healthier community

Take a moment to share your journey and lead someone to a life-changing discovery. Leave a review today and be part of the wellness revolution by scanning the QR code below or visiting https://rb.gy/p18asb.

With gratitude,
Dr. Cynthia McCallister

# 15. Sauna-based Cardiovascular Endurance Training
## A Strategy to Prevent Disease, Promote Healing, and Enhance Health and Well-being

Pursuing optimal health and longevity has led humans to investigate numerous approaches for preventing disease and enhancing overall well-being. Among these strategies, exercise—particularly cardiovascular endurance training (CET)—has emerged as one of the most effective methods for improving health outcomes and potentially extending lifespan.

One of the most transformative approaches to sauna practice is *sauna-based cardiovascular endurance training* (S-CET), which challenges you to gradually build your heat tolerance over time to reap the enormous health benefits of heat stress on all the body's systems. By alternating periods of intense heat with cool-down showers, you are essentially conducting a controlled way of stressing your body, using heat as a source of hormesis, and stimulating the physiological processes that underly health and well-being described in the previous section of the book. This process of progressive adaptation is a powerful metaphor for how we can grow and evolve as individuals when we embrace discomfort and challenge ourselves to reach new heights.

This chapter delves into the foundational principles that explain the power of cardiovascular endurance training and how sauna practice offers a strategy that individuals of any age or fitness level can use to develop cardiovascular fitness and reap the vast benefits of health and well-being. We begin by discussing the benefits of CET and the promise of S-CET as an alternative. We then review some fundamental principles of CET before delving into protocols for S-CET.

**Benefits of Cardiovascular Endurance Training**

CET is highly beneficial to health due to its profound and multifaceted impact, with the most fundamental effect being improving cardiovascular function and metabolic efficiency. This exercise strengthens the heart muscle, enhances blood circulation, and increases lung capacity, allowing for more efficient oxygen delivery. These improvements lead to better overall endurance, reduced risk of heart disease, and enhanced cellular metabolism. Regular cardiovascular activity helps maintain a healthy weight, regulates blood pressure, improves cholesterol levels, and aids in better blood sugar control, making it beneficial for managing diabetes. Beyond physical health, it positively affects mental well-being by stimulating the release of endorphins and other beneficial hormones, which reduce stress and anxiety. CET positively impacts nearly every aspect of physical and mental health, from improved immune function to better cognitive performance. Ultimately, regular CET training is linked to increased longevity, effectively improving both the quality and quantity of life.

**Sauna as an Alternative to Muscular Cardiovascular Exercise**

Conventional wisdom has long held that elevating heart rate through physical exertion is the primary path to enhancing heart health and endurance. Traditional CET typically involves muscular activities like running, cycling, or swimming.

Emerging research suggests that heat stress on the body experienced during the sauna may offer a promising alternative for improving cardiovascular fitness. This more passive form of stress on the cardiovascular system, induced by high temperatures rather than physical activity, triggers adaptations similar to traditional muscular exercise. The sauna also provides a low-impact way to get your heart rate up without the physical pounding and stress of activities like running, making rigorous cardio exercise available to anyone, regardless of physical limitations.

This chapter provides an overview of how sauna training can be harnessed as a powerful tool in pursuing optimal health and resilience against disease, offering a new perspective on cardiovascular condition-ing. It begins with an overview of the physiological effects and benefits of CET training. It then describes protocols for what we refer to as S-CET, in which periods of heat exposure are done in alternating intervals with cold showers as a strategy to increase the strength of the cardiovas-cular-respiratory system, to improve the volume of oxygen that can be used during exercise, to induce the expression of heat shock proteins (HSPs) by elevating the heart rate, and to strengthen the parasympa-thetic nervous system.

**Cardio-training: Physiology Fundamentals**

Cardiovascular endurance training (CET) involves structured aerobic exercises that challenge and improve the heart, lungs, and circu-latory system in response to the body's demand for oxygen. The objec-tive of the training is to increase the maximum rate at which the body can utilize oxygen during intense activity, symbolized as ↑VO2 max.

*VO2 max: Maximal oxygen uptake*

VO2 max, also known as maximal oxygen uptake, is the maximum rate at which an individual can transport and utilize oxygen during intense exercise and is considered one of the best indicators of cardiovas-cular fitness and aerobic endurance. A high VO2 max is associated with improved overall health and longevity. Studies have shown that individ-uals with higher VO2 max values have a lower risk of cardiovascular disease, obesity, and all-cause mortality. Research suggests that for every 3.5 ml/kg/min increase in VO2max, there is a 13% reduction in all-cause mortality risk.

The impact of increased oxygen uptake through training becomes more evident when we examine the numbers. An average person's heart pumps about 2.5 ounces of blood per beat, or, at 75 beats per minute, a gallon and a half of blood per minute. An elite athlete's heart can pump up to 3.5 ounces per beat with a larger stroke volume. This seemingly small difference adds up dramatically over time. An elite athlete's body may circulate an extra half gallon of blood in just one minute compared to an average person. Consider that a gallon of blood carries about 756 ml (or 25 ounces) of oxygen—roughly the volume of a wine bottle or 3 cups. With superior cardiovascular effi-ciency, elite athletes can process up to 2 gallons of blood per minute, delivering a staggering 1.5 liters of oxygen—equivalent to a quart and a half.

This increased circulation and oxygen delivery enhances cellular respiration and energy production throughout the body, improving overall metabolic function. Additionally, it promotes better tissue oxygenation, which can aid in recovery, reduce inflammation, support immune function, and potentially improve cognitive performance. Over time, this consistent blood flow and oxygen delivery increase can improve cardiovascular health, endurance, and overall physical and mental well-being.

### Cardiac output

Cardiac output is the volume of blood pumped by the heart per minute, typically measured in liters per minute. It is calculated by multiplying stroke volume (blood pumped per beat) by heart rate.

Cardiac output plays a pivotal role in determining VO2 max. As exercise intensity increases, heart rate and stroke volume rise, resulting in higher cardiac output. This increased cardiac output is crucial for delivering oxygen to working muscles during exercise. VO2 max is dependent mainly on this cardiac output.

The Fick equation describes the relationship between cardiac output and VO2 max: VO2 = Cardiac Output × (a-vO2 difference), where a-vO2 represents the amount of oxygen the tissues extract.

During maximal exercise, cardiac output can increase dramatically, up to five or six times its resting value in untrained individuals and up to eight times in elite athletes. Over time, with training, the heart can pump more as the size of the heart's left ventricle increases in volume, and more oxygen can be extracted by the tissues as capillary density or the number of capillaries in a given area of the skin increases. Consequently, improvements in cardiac output through endurance training, primarily via increases in stroke volume and capillary density, are a key mechanism for enhancing VO2 max and overall aerobic capacity. These processes are explained below.

### Stroke volume

When the body is subjected to intense heat or physical exercise, the heart muscle (myocardium) strengthens, and the left ventricle volume expands. This enlargement allows the heart to pump more blood with each stroke. This phenomenon is known as the Frank-Starling Mechanism, which states that the heart's stroke volume increases in response to an increase in the volume of blood filling the heart (the end-diastolic volume) when all other factors remain constant. The increased amount of blood flowing back from the veins into the heart—venous return—stretches the ventricular walls, causing cardiac muscle fibers to contract more forcefully.

Through cardio training and the increased volume of the left ventricle, athletes can increase their heart's efficiency, pumping 40% more blood per beat than the average person. This improved efficiency means their hearts work significantly less over time. In an 80-year lifespan, while an average heart might beat 3 billion times, an athlete's heart could beat 1.2 billion times fewer—only 1.8 billion beats total. This reduced workload potentially contributes to improved cardiovascular health and longevity.

### Capillary density

In response to increased demands for oxygen during training, the body promotes the formation of new *capillaries*, a process known as *angiogenesis*, leading to higher *capillary density*. Higher capillary density allows for better perfusion of tissues, ensuring that cells receive an adequate supply of oxygen and nutrients necessary for their proper function and survival. Additionally, capillaries help remove metabolic waste products, such as carbon dioxide and lactic acid, from the tissues, and higher capillary density facilitates more efficient removal of these waste products, preventing their accumulation and potential damage to cells. Capillaries also contribute to thermoregulation by providing a greater surface area for heat exchange when capillary density increases, allowing the body to dissipate heat and maintain a stable core temperature more effectively.

### Increased plasma volume

CET training can lead to an increase in *plasma volume*. Increased plasma volume is a significant adaptation to endurance exercise. This increase occurs both acutely after individual exercise sessions and chronically with consistent training over time. When the body is exposed to the stress of training, blood vessels dilate, causing a fluid shift from the blood plasma to the interstitial space or the space between cells and tissues. Increased plasma production compensates for this fluid shift and maintains blood pressure. This increase in plasma volume helps maintain proper cardiovascular function. It offers potential benefits such as improved cardiovascular endurance, enhanced venous return, increased stroke volume, improved thermoregulation during exercise, and potential performance benefits for athletes.

Regular CET training can result in plasma volume expansions of 10-20% in well-trained individuals compared to sedentary controls. This adaptation is one reason endurance athletes often display lower hematocrit levels, or percentage of red blood cells in a given blood volume, despite having normal or elevated total red blood cell mass, as the increased plasma effectively dilutes the blood. Increased plasma volume is a key physiological response that improves cardiovascular performance and exercise capacity.

**Training Principles**

Regular aerobic exercise can improve VO2 max by enhancing the body's ability to deliver oxygen to tissues and improving their efficiency in utilizing oxygen. The primary aim of training is to bring more oxygen into the body. An activity that raises the heart rate by 40 beats per minute over 30 minutes brings 23 additional gallons of blood into the body and about 4.5 gallons of oxygen.

To continue seeing improvements in VO2 max, the intensity, duration, or frequency of training over time must gradually increase. This principle, known as *progressive overload*, ensures that the body is continually challenged and adapts to the increasing demands. Once a high level of VO2 max has been achieved, regular training is necessary to maintain it. Detraining, or the cessation of regular exercise, can decrease VO2 max over time.

High-intensity training, particularly high-intensity interval training (HIIT), effectively improves VO2max. HIIT involves short bursts of intense exercise followed by periods of rest or low-intensity exercise. This training is the most rigorous way to challenge the cardiovascular system and can lead to greater improvements in VO2 max compared to moderate-intensity continuous training.

The American College of Sports Medicine recommends 150 minutes of moderate-intensity or 75 minutes of vigorous-intensity aerobic exercise per week for general health. However, to significantly improve VO2 max, individuals may need to engage in more frequent and prolonged training sessions. Training should be specific to the individual's goals and the demands of their chosen sport or activity. For example, a long-distance runner would benefit from training emphasizing longer, sustained efforts. At the same time, a soccer player might focus on shorter, high-intensity intervals to mimic the demands of the game.

By engaging in a regular, well-designed training program that incorporates aerobic exercise and progressive overload, individuals can improve their VO2 max and overall aerobic fitness. While VO2 max can be improved through traditional physical exercise, heat from the sauna can be used as a training strategy to increase VO2 max.

### Understanding Your Heart Rate

Heart rate, the number of times your heart beats per minute (bpm), is an essential indicator of cardiovascular health and fitness. Various factors influence your heart rate, including physical activity, stress, hormones, and overall health. However, heart rate is often used in physical fitness to gauge exercise intensity and monitor cardiovascular health improvements.

There are several key levels of heart rate relevant to physical fitness:

### *Resting heart rate (RHR)*

Resting heart rate (RHR) is your heart rate at rest, typically measured when you wake up before engaging in physical activity. A lower RHR generally indicates better cardiovascular fitness, as the heart doesn't have to work as hard to pump blood.

### *Maximum heart rate (MHR)*

Maximum heart rate (MHR) is the maximum number of times your heart can beat in one minute during intense exercise. The most common estimation of MHR is 220 minus your age, though this is a rough estimate and varies from person to person.

### *Heart rate zones*

Heart rate zones are a way to measure the intensity of your cardiovascular exercise based on your heart rate during the activity. These zones are determined by your maximum heart rate (MHR), the highest number of times your heart can beat in one minute. You can target specific fitness goals and optimize your workouts by training in different heart rate zones.

Target Heart Rate (THR) Zones are the heart rate ranges within which you should aim to exercise to achieve specific fitness goals. Zones commonly used to gauge exercise intensity range from 1 to 5. Remember that these are general guidelines, and your needs may vary based on your fitness level, health status, and workout goals. If you're new to heart rate training or have any medical concerns, consult a healthcare professional or certified fitness trainer to determine the most appropriate heart rate zones and monitoring frequency. Especially when you begin, it's essential to pay close attention to your heart rate to avoid overexertion and potential health risks. The heat in a sauna can cause your heart rate to increase quickly and significantly as your body works to regulate its internal temperature through vasodilation and increased blood flow to the skin.

### *Monitoring your heart rate during training*

Monitoring your heart rate during exercise can help you stay within your target zones and optimize the effectiveness of your workouts. Over time, as you improve your cardiovascular fitness, you may find that your heart rate is lower at given exercise intensities, indicating improved efficiency of your heart and circulatory system.

Taking your pulse is a simple way to measure your heart rate without using electronic devices, which can't withstand the high temperature of the sauna. To take your pulse, follow these steps:

1. *Find your pulse:* You can find your pulse on your wrist (radial artery) or neck (carotid artery).

For the wrist, use your index and middle fingers to feel the pulse on the inside of your wrist, just below the base of your thumb.

Use your index and middle fingers for the neck to feel the pulse on either side of your windpipe, just below your jawline.

2. *Count the beats:* Once you've located your pulse, count the number of beats you feel within a specific time frame.

For a 15-second count, multiply beats by 4 to get your heart rate in beats per minute (bpm).

For a 30-second count, multiply the beats by 2 to get your heart rate in bpm.

*3. Assess your heart rate:* Compare your measured heart rate to your target range to ensure you're not overexerting during the sauna session.

While an elevated heart rate is a normal response to the sauna environment, monitoring it to avoid overexertion and potential health risks is crucial. If you have a pre-existing heart condition or are taking medications that affect your heart rate, consult with your healthcare provider before starting a sauna routine and follow their guidance on safe heart rate limits.

If you notice that your heart rate is consistently exceeding your target range or if you experience symptoms such as dizziness, lightheadedness, or chest discomfort, it's important to exit the sauna immediately and allow your body to cool down. Taking breaks between sauna rounds, staying hydrated, and listening to your body's signals are all crucial aspects of a safe and enjoyable sauna routine.

By monitoring your heart rate and respecting your body's limits, you can maximize the potential health benefits of sauna while minimizing the risk of adverse effects on your cardiovascular system.

**The Relationship Between Exercise and Heat Shock Protein Expression**

The intricate relationship between exercise intensity zones and heat shock protein (HSP) expression represents a fascinating intersection of exercise physiology and cellular biology. As we push our bodies through various levels of physical exertion, from low-intensity steady-state activities to high-intensity interval training, we trigger a cascade of molecular responses designed to protect and adapt our cells.

As you recall, heat shock proteins (HSPs) are a family of molecular chaperones induced by various stressors, including heat and physical strain, that play a pivotal role in cellular protection and reversing disease processes, making them a key factor in the therapeutic benefits of sauna use. The expression of HSPs is closely related to the intensity of the stressor, which can be linked to the heart rate zones. As heart rate increases during exercise or stress, body temperature rises, triggering the production of HSPs. Heart rate and heat shock proteins (HSPs) are linked through the body's stress response mechanisms.

Heat shock proteins play a crucial role in this adaptive process. This section explores how different exercise intensity zones influence the expression of HSPs, offering insights into the mechanisms by which our bodies respond to and benefit from diverse training stimuli. Understanding this relationship deepens our knowledge of exercise-induced adaptations and provides valuable information for optimizing training protocols and potentially enhancing health outcomes. In the section below, we review the relationship between HR and HSPs at every level of physical exercise intensity.

### *Resting heart rate and HSPs*

Resting Heart Rate (RHR) is your heart rate when you're at rest and not performing any physical activity. A typical adult RHR ranges from 60 to 100 bpm, but it can be lower for athletes or people with high cardiovascular fitness. *Safety:* This zone is your natural state, where your heart is safely beating. There is no need to check your pulse in this zone unless you have a medical condition that requires monitoring.

*HSP expression at RHR*

At basal levels, the body's energy systems operate at baseline levels and under no significant stress that would trigger increased HSP synthesis. At resting heart rate, HSPs play roles in protein folding, transport, and quality control, helping to maintain cellular homeostasis.

*Zone 1: HSPs and very light-intensity exercise (less than 57% of MHR)*

Low-intensity exercise is used for warm-up, cool-down, and recovery exercises. It's ideal for beginners or those with health concerns.

- *Safety:* Zone 1 exercise is safe for extended periods, even several hours. You don't need to check your pulse frequently in this zone, perhaps once every 10-15 minutes.
- *Zone 1 HSP expression:* HSP is minimal or not significantly elevated in this zone. The body is under very little stress, and cells aren't experiencing significant heat or other stressors that would trigger HSP production. This activity level is generally too low to stimulate meaningful adaptations in the body's stress response systems.

*Zone 2: HSPs and light-intensity exercise (57-63% of MHR)*
In light-intensity exercise, the body primarily burns fat for fuel. Its

moderate intensity level is suitable for longer-duration workouts, such as steady-state cardio or walking.

- *Safety:* Zone 2 exercise is safe for prolonged periods, typically 60 minutes or more. You should check your pulse every 10 minutes to make sure you stay within the target range.
- *Zone 2 HSP expression:* HSP production increases slightly in this zone, becoming more pronounced as the exercise continues. During Zone 2 exercise, the body experiences mild physiological stress, including a slight increase in core temperature and oxidative stress. As the body's temperature rises marginally and cells experience mild metabolic stress, there's a slight uptick in HSP synthesis, protecting cells from exercise-induced stress, aiding in protein folding, and contributing to cellular adaptation to regular exercise. While the response is still relatively low, and significant adaptations are unlikely to occur at this light intensity, the increased HSP expression can contribute to cardioprotective effects, helping the heart adapt to stress. And even while the HSP response in Zone 2 exercise isn't as pronounced as in high-intensity exercise or heat shock, the consistent, long-duration nature of Zone 2 training can lead to cumulative benefits in terms of HSP-mediated cellular protection and adaptation over time.

*Zone 3: HSPs and vigorous-intensity exercise (64-76% of MHR)*

Exercise in the vigorous intensity zone is moderate to high intensity and helps increase aerobic capacity, cardiovascular fitness, and endurance.

- *Safety:* Zone 3 exercise is safe for 30 to 60 minutes per session and is recommended for most people seeking to maintain or improve their fitness level. Check your pulse every 5-7 minutes to maintain the desired intensity.

- *Zone 3 HSP expression:* HSP expression significantly amplifies compared to rest or light activity. The increased intensity increases body temperature and greater cellular stress, triggering a more substantial HSP response in the heart, skeletal muscles, and other organs. Over time, regular vigorous exercise is sufficient to stimulate adaptations in the body's stress response systems. This leads to higher baseline HSP levels, enhances the body's overall stress resistance, and improves exercise performance and health benefits.

### Zone 4: HSPs and high-intensity exercise (77-95% of MHR)

This high-intensity zone is used for interval training and improving anaerobic capacity. It's effective for improving speed and power but should be approached with caution due to its intensity. High-intensity exercise is used for high-intensity interval training (HIIT). It helps improve cardiovascular fitness and increases lactate threshold. It should only be performed by individuals with a solid fitness base.

- *Safety:* High-intensity exercise is safe for 10 minutes to 30 minutes per session. Check your pulse every 3-5 minutes, as you may need to adjust your effort more frequently to stay within the zone.
- *Zone 4 HSP expression:* HSP expression is significantly elevated in this zone due to the high-intensity nature of the exercise, which causes considerable heat stress and metabolic demands on cells. This activity level can significantly increase cellular protection and adaptation, improving stress resilience and performance.

### Zone 5: HSPs and maximal-intensity (96-100% of MHR)

You push your heart to its absolute limit in the maximum effort zone. It's typically used for short burst speed training or high-intensity exercise and should be approached cautiously to avoid injury or overexertion. Elite athletes use it for very high-intensity exercises, and it's not recommended for beginners or individuals with underlying health conditions.

- *Safety:* Maximal-intensity exercise is only safe for short durations, typically less than 5 minutes at a time. During maximal intensity exercise, focus on maintaining intensity briefly rather than checking your pulse. If you need to check, do so every 1-2 minutes.
- *Zone 5 HSP expression:* The extreme stress placed on the body at near-maximal intensity triggers a robust HSP response in cells to prevent cellular damage and maintain homeostasis. While this can lead to significant adaptations, the intensity is typically sustainable only for short periods due to the high stress level.

**Sauna-based Interval Training: Alternating Heat and Cold Exposure**

Exposure to intense heat is a potential strategy to improve cardiac capacity and VO2 max and to increase HSP expression. During a sauna session, the extreme heat causes blood vessels near the skin to dilate, increasing cardiac output and heart rate as your body warms.

After the body has begun to sweat and the heart rate rises, a 15-20-minute sauna session at around 160-195°F (70-90°C) can raise the heart rate by 50-75% above resting levels, similar to moderate-intensity exercise. With more time in the heat, the heart rate increases in intensity until it's working at maximal intensity.

The rapid heart rate provoked by the sauna heat initiates the first training interval. After achieving a target heart rate and maintaining it for the desired period, cooling off with a cold shower for 1-3 minutes dramatically lowers the skin's surface temperature, causing the superficial blood vessels to constrict quickly and reducing the heart rate. The interval concludes with the cooling-off period. In subsequent intervals, the heart rate can be strategically raised and lowered by alternating between hot sauna sessions and cold showers.

Stacking heat and cold exposure in intervals strengthens the heart and circulatory system like other forms of interval training, such as HIIT, which involves short bursts of intense exercise followed by rest periods. The length and number of intervals can be adjusted according to the goals of your training program. By deliberately manipulating your heart rate to alter between heat-induced elevation and cold-induced recovery periods, you give your heart and circulatory system a targeted workout while enjoying the other health benefits of sauna therapy described in the previous section of the book.

### Physiology of S-CET

The body makes physiological adaptations in S-CET that are stimulated by high and low-temperature extremes but in different ways.

*High-temperature exposure*

through repeated exposure to heat stress, such as those described above, such as increasing plasma, improving cardiovascular function, and enhancing oxygen delivery, which can increase VO2 max. The effects can be significant. In a study by Lorenzo and colleagues (2010), heat adaptation significantly increased VO2 max. This research involved 20 experienced cyclists. The participants were divided into two groups: one trained in a hot environment, while the other trained in a cool setting. Before beginning a 10-day training regimen, researchers measured various aerobic parameters for all cyclists. These measurements were repeated at the conclusion of the training period. The results were remarkable. The group that adapted to heat showed significant improvements in just ten days. Their VO2 max (maximum oxygen uptake) increased by 8% in hot and 5% in cool conditions. They demonstrated a 5% increase in power output at the lactate threshold, regardless of whether they were in hot or cool environments. These findings suggest that heat acclimatization training can lead to substantial performance enhancements in a relatively short time, with benefits extending to both hot and cool conditions.

*Low-temperature exposure*

The cooling process in the S-CET brings about another set of benefits. In rapid cooling, blood is forced back into the inner body, exerting increased pressure in the capillaries. The movement between expansion and constriction in S-CET improves capillary compliance or the ability of the cells to expand or distend in response to changes in blood pressure or blood volume. It measures how easily these tiny vessels can accommodate changes in blood flow and pressure.

Rapid cooling also activates Brown Adipose Tissue (BAT), triggering a process called non-shivering thermogenesis described previously. This activation increases BAT's metabolic activity, as BAT burns more glucose and fatty acids, generating heat to maintain core body temperature. This process enhances glucose uptake and fatty acid oxidation, potentially improving insulin sensitivity and lipid metabolism. Regular cold exposure can lead to BAT recruitment, increasing the body's capacity for thermogenesis. It also stimulates norepinephrine release, further activating BAT. As more blood is forced into the cells of the inner body, the production of energy increases in the cells, where the strength of the mitochondria improves, and new mitochondria grow. These effects collectively improve metabolic health and may aid in weight management.

The magnitude of the cooling effect experienced during cold exposure is related to the amount of energy or oxygen moving through the body's system. While exposure in any condition triggers a cascade of positive physiological responses, the impact is significantly amplified when performed immediately after a high-intensity sauna session. In this scenario, the body is already in a state of heightened metabolic activity, with increased blood flow and oxygen circulation. When suddenly exposed to cold, this energized system responds exponentially more intensely. The contrast between the sauna-induced heat stress and the rapid cooling creates a more pronounced thermal shock, leading to a more powerful activation of brown adipose tissue, a stronger cardiovascular response, and potentially greater benefits in recovery, circulation, and overall metabolic boost. This synergistic effect of heat followed by cold maximizes the body's adaptive responses, potentially offering enhanced health benefits compared to cold exposure alone.

### Recruiting Heat Shock Proteins in Sauna-based Interval Training for Therapeutic Effects

Strategically manipulating the heart rate through S-CET increases the body's expression of HSPs, harnessing their protective and therapeutic properties and aiding in preventing and reversing numerous disease processes discussed in the previous book section. If you aim to prevent or reverse disease processes, your objective might be to train your body to tolerate heat of a length and intensity that results in optimal HSP expression.

Skillful modulation of cardiovascular activity through S-CET enhances the body's production of Heat Shock Proteins (HSPs), unlocking their potent protective and restorative capabilities. As explored in previous chapters, HSPs play a powerful role in preventing and reversing myriad disease processes. For those seeking to fortify their defenses against illness or initiate cellular repair, the goal becomes clear: cultivating the body's resilience to heat and carefully calibrating the duration and intensity of exposure to elicit optimal HSP expression. This strategic approach to thermal stress bolsters the body's innate healing mechanisms. It lays the groundwork for sustained vitality and longevity, offering a sophisticated means to harness the body's protective resources to pursue holistic health.

It's important to note that while HSP expression is a natural stress response and can be beneficial in moderation, prolonged exposure to high-intensity stress (such as spending too much time in the Hard and Maximum zones) can lead to overexpression of HSPs, which may be detrimental to overall health. Always allow adequate recovery or cooldown time between high-intensity intervals and workouts, and listen to your body to avoid overtraining. The next chapter outlines a graduated approach to S-CET training that can be used to train your body to withstand increasing levels of heat safely.

### Sauna-based Cardiovascular Endurance Training to Strengthen the Parasympathetic Nervous System

Sauna interval training presents an innovative approach to strengthening the parasympathetic nervous system. It offers a unique blend of heat stress and controlled recovery that can significantly impact our body's ability to relax and regenerate. This section explores the intriguing concept of using structured sauna sessions to enhance the parasympathetic tone.

The physical discomfort experienced in higher exercise intensity zones (Zone 2 and above) offers a unique opportunity to observe and modulate the mind's response to stress. By consciously overriding the acute stress and the urge to flee, we can train our minds to activate the parasympathetic nervous system—often called the "rest and digest" or relaxation response—even under challenging conditions. Deliberately maintaining composure during heat stress that elevates cardiac output to Zones 3-4 can yield effects comparable to established parasympathetic stimulation techniques, such as deep breathing, mindfulness meditation, progressive muscle relaxation, yin yoga, or guided imagery. This practice enhances physical endurance and cultivates mental resilience and autonomic balance, potentially improving stress management in various life situations.

So, instead of giving in to the natural impulse to exit the sauna when discomfort sets in, observe their mind's reaction to the stress and try not to react. These opportunities can train the mind to remain calm in physical stress. This approach essentially combines high-intensity exercise with mindfulness practices, potentially offering a powerful method for improving both physical fitness and mental well-being. It teaches the body and mind to remain calm and composed even under significant physical stress, which can translate to better stress management in everyday life. Moreover, this practice may help improve overall exercise performance by training yourself to push through discomfort more effectively, potentially leading to greater endurance and higher-intensity workouts.

### Advantages of Sauna-based Cardiovascular Endurance Training

Sauna-based cardiovascular endurance training (S-CET) offers several advantages over traditional, muscular cardio training due to the skin's unique properties compared to muscles.

Passive physical conditioning using the thermoregulatory process has unique advantages over physical conditioning involving the muscles. The muscles account for 30-45% of body weight, more than double that of the skin. Muscles are responsible for generating force and require significant energy (ATP) to contract and generate force. This process can lead to fatigue when energy stores are depleted. Muscle fibers can experience micro-tears and damage during intense or prolonged activity, contributing to fatigue and requiring time for repair and recovery. The skin's primary functions do not involve generating force or movement. Its rich blood supply provides adequate oxygen and nutrients to maintain its function without causing fatigue. It has a regenerative capacity, with cells constantly undergoing division and replacement to maintain the skin's integrity without experiencing fatigue.

Here's how thermoregulatory cardio training in the sauna avoids some of the limitations of muscular cardio training:

### Fatigue resistance

Muscles are prone to fatigue due to lactic acid buildup during intense or prolonged exercise. Lactic acid is a byproduct of anaerobic metabolism and can cause muscle soreness, reduced performance, and the need for recovery time. In contrast, skin does not produce lactic acid during heat therapy, allowing for longer duration and more consistent cardiovascular stress without the limitations of muscle fatigue.

### Continuous cardiovascular stress

During muscular cardio training, the cardiovascular system experiences intermittent stress as muscles alternate between contraction and relaxation. This can lead to fluctuations in heart rate and blood flow. Heat therapy, on the other hand, provides more continuous and stable cardiovascular stress by consistently stimulating the skin's blood vessels and promoting blood flow. This sustained cardiovascular challenge can lead to improved endurance and cardiovascular adaptations.

### Systemic effect

Muscular cardio training primarily targets specific muscle groups involved in the exercise, such as the legs, during running or cycling. While this can lead to localized adaptations, heat therapy has a more systemic effect on the body. When the skin is exposed to heat, blood vessels throughout the body dilate, increasing overall blood flow and cardiovascular demand. This systemic response can lead to improved vascular function and cardiovascular health.

### Accessibility and compliance

Muscular cardio training often requires specific equipment, facilities, or outdoor spaces, limiting accessibility for some individuals. Heat therapy can be performed using various methods, such as saunas, hot baths, or heated garments, making it more accessible and convenient. Heat therapy sessions can also be easily incorporated into daily routines, potentially increasing compliance compared to structured exercise programs.

S-CET has additional advantages for frail and elderly individuals:

### Passive form of stress

One key advantage of heat therapy for elderly and frail individuals is its passive nature. Unlike active muscular cardio training, which requires physical exertion and can be challenging for those with limited mobility or strength, heat therapy allows cardiovascular benefits without requiring active movement. Its passive nature makes it an ideal option for elderly and frail individuals with physical limitations preventing them from engaging in traditional cardio exercises.

### Reduced risk of injury

For elderly and frail individuals who are more susceptible to injuries during physical activities due to reduced muscle mass, decreased bone density, and impaired balance, heat therapy minimizes the risk of injury as it does not involve weight-bearing activities or high-impact movements. The more passive nature of heat exposure makes it a safer alternative for those at a higher risk of falls or musculoskeletal injuries.

### Improved circulation

Elderly and frail individuals often experience reduced circulation due to age-related changes in the cardiovascular system. Heat therapy can help improve circulation by dilating blood vessels and promoting blood flow throughout the body. This enhanced circulation can contribute to better overall cardiovascular health, oxygenation of tissues, and nutrient delivery.

### Stress reduction and relaxation

Heat therapy can provide a relaxing and stress-reducing effect. The warmth and comfort associated with heat exposure can promote a sense of well-being, reduce anxiety, and improve sleep quality. These psychological benefits can positively impact overall health and quality of life.

It's important to note that while heat therapy offers unique benefits, it should not be seen as a complete replacement for muscular cardio training. Muscular cardio training can provide additional benefits, such as improved muscle strength, bone density, and overall functional capacity when performed safely and under proper guidance. Ideally, a well-rounded cardiovascular training program would incorporate heat therapy and appropriate muscular cardio exercises tailored to the individual's needs and abilities.

### Conclusion

In conclusion, sauna-based cardiovascular endurance training (S-CET) offers a powerful and accessible approach to enhancing health and longevity. By alternating between intense heat exposure and rapid cooling, S-CET mimics the benefits of traditional cardiovascular exercise while providing unique advantages. This method improves cardiovascular fitness, VO2 max, and metabolic efficiency while harnessing the body's adaptive responses to thermal stress, particularly through heat shock protein expression. S-CET's low-impact nature makes it suitable for individuals of varying fitness levels, offering a way to optimize protective and therapeutic processes. As a synthesis of ancient wisdom and modern science, S-CET is a promising tool for cultivating resilience, vitality, and longevity through controlled thermal stress.

# 16. Training the Music of Your Heart

Think of the heart's beating as the tempo of your bodily systems, and imagine your heart as the conductor who guides the tempo of the symphony of energy within your body. Just as a conductor guides an orchestra, your heart orchestrates the flow of energy throughout your entire being.

In music, composers use specific terms called *tempo markings* to dictate the pace of a piece. Tempo markings, displayed below, offer an intuitive framework for understanding the heart's various rhythms, allowing us to conceptualize how changes in heart rate—from the slow adagio of rest to the vivace of exertion—reflect and influence our body's overall state and energy levels.

- Larghissimo: Under 20 BPM
- Grave: 20-40 BPM
- Lento: 40-60 BPM
- Largo: 40-60 BPM
- Adagio: 66-76 BPM
- Andante: 76-108 BPM
- Moderato: 108-120 BPM

- Allegretto: 112-120 BPM
- Allegro: 120-168 BPM
- Vivace: 168-176 BPM
- Presto: 168-200 BPM
- Prestissimo: Over 200 BPM

The tempo of a weak heart is like an inconsistent musical performance. Unlike a healthy heart's steady, adaptable rhythm, a weak heart may struggle to maintain a regular beat, with the need to beat too quickly (tachycardia). Once exerted, the heart might struggle to return to a normal rate, indicating that the cardiovascular system has difficulty reaching its resting condition efficiently. This weaker "performance" results in a narrow dynamic range, with unpredictable arrhythmic patterns disrupting the symphony of blood circulation in the body.

Those with strong hearts can push them to perform in rapid-tempo zones and to quickly and easily transition between tempos. At rest, the well-trained heart can play a calm Adagio, effortlessly transition to a vigorous Allegro during exercise, and gracefully descend back to its resting beat. It can adapt its tempo to meet the body's changing demands, maintaining a robust and consistent rhythm that orchestrates energy flow.

Just as a composer controls the tempo of a piece of music, you can control and change the tempo of the music of your heart through sauna interval training.

This chapter will guide you in embarking on a journey of practice to improve the music of your heart. I began by sharing insights form my practice, then offer recommendations for you to improve the music of your heart.

### My Journey of the Heart

When I began my sauna journey and struggled with nervous system dysregulation, the tempo of my resting heart rate was over 100, which posed certain health risks. Higher resting heart rates are linked to increased mortality risk. Over time, consistently elevated heart rates can strain the heart, possibly leading to cardiovascular problems. Each increase of ten beats per minute potentially raises the risk of death from all causes by 9-16%.

I've strengthened my heart's performance through three years of sauna training. Each day, I play the music of my heart in tune with my body's mood and energy level. When energized, I can play fast and intense music, like the workout presented below, where my heart reaches its crescendo in the maximal zone once in each of the three intervals.

- 4:20 pm: Begin sauna session sitting upright
- 4:35 pm: Achieved profuse sweating
- 4:45 pm: Laid down after achieving a heart rate of 120 (Borderline between Zone 2 and 3)
- 5:05 pm: Sat up to raise heart rate
- 5:10 pm: Achieved heart rate of 152, reaching the maximal zone
- Break: 1 minute standing, 1 minute sitting, 1 minute cold shower, 1 minute sitting until achieving a heart rate of 104
- 5:15 pm: Re-entered sauna, laid down
- 5:30 pm: Sat up until achieving a heart rate of 160 (Zone 5)
- Break to cool down: 1-minute standing, 1-minute sitting, 1-minute cold shower, 1-minute sitting, until achieving a heart rate of 100
- 5:40 pm: Re-entered sauna, laid down
- 5:45 pm: Sat up until achieving a heart rate of 140 (zone 4)
- 5:50 pm: Exited sauna. 5-minute cold shower.

Described as a piece of music in the workout played above, I began in Adagio at 70 beats per minute. I let my heart rate climb through Andante to achieve Moderato for an extended interval before sitting up to achieve Allegro for several minutes, reaching 152 beats per minute. After a cooling refrain, I began another movement in Andante, and the piece continued through another two intervals or *movements*. The music structure for this sauna workout could be described as A-B-C-D-B-C-D-B-C-D-A, where A is my resting heart rate, B is zone 2, C is zone 3, and D is zone 4-5.

I do a slow workout on days I don't feel like playing at rapid tempos. I spend most of the time lying on my back with my heart in Moderato, beating at 110. I sit up briefly to bring it to 120-130 before cooling down before the next interval. The structure of the music for slower workouts is something like this: A-B-C- B-C- B-C-A.

With consistent practice, I've trained my heart to shift tempos effortlessly throughout a typical sauna session. I once had tachycardia, with a resting heart rate above 100. My heart is now stronger, with a resting pace of 67. Lowering my heart rate has significant positive implications for my mortality risk. A large-scale study conducted in Taiwan examined the relationship between resting heart rate (RHR) and mortality risk among 515,303 adults (Chen et al., 2017). The research revealed a significant association between elevated RHR and increased mortality. Notably, individuals with an RHR between 80-99 beats per minute (bpm) had a 40% shorter lifespan than those with an RHR of 60–69 bpm.

I think of the sauna as daily training for the music of my heart, so I might relish the joy of listening for a long time to come.

**Structuring A Sauna-based Cardiovascular Endurance Training Program: From Beginner to Advanced**

Utilizing sauna sessions for cardiovascular endurance training offers a unique and potentially powerful approach to enhancing overall health and well-being, combining the physiological stress of heat exposure with traditional endurance training methods. By leveraging the body's adaptive responses to heat stress and cardiovascular exercise, this approach aims to amplify the benefits typically associated with endurance training alone.

In a well-structured cardiovascular training program, the proportion of time spent in each heart rate zone depends on your fitness level, goals, and the specific training phase you are in. However, a general guideline for most individuals is to focus primarily on Zone 2 training, with a smaller proportion of higher-intensity work in Zones 3 and 4, depending on overall cardiovascular fitness. The following three sections explore principles for structuring such a training program. It will guide you through the practical aspects of designing such a program, including considerations for timing, frequency, and intensity of sauna use about endurance workouts.

### Beginner level

Start slowly if you're a beginner and new to sauna practice and cardio training. If you have a health condition, get approval from your healthcare provider to begin sauna practice. Then, clarify your goals. If you want to improve cardiovascular fitness, you might, for example, plan to visit the sauna three times a week for 15 minutes a day to get accustomed to the hot environment and to learn to read your body.

Take your pulse every few minutes to gauge your body's response to the heat. Let your heart play music in an A-B-C-B-C-A structure (resting heart rate to zone 1 heart rate to zone 2 heart rate, to zone 1 heart rate, to zone 2 heart rate, then cool off to resting heart rate).

Once you're accustomed to the environment and know the music of your heart, increase the number of days you practice, the number of intervals in your practice, and the length of each session. With sustained practice, as your heart grows stronger, you can tolerate longer durations of more heat. You might add an interval so your workout will play a piece in an A-B-C-B-C-A structure. See the sample beginner routine below.

*Beginner routine*

Two intervals for a total of 20 minutes on the bottom shelf of a 185° sauna

*Interval 1*

5-minutes sitting up, warming up to open capillaries, begin sweating, and reaching zone 2 heart rate

5-minutes lying down, maintaining zone 2-3 heart rate

1-minute sitting up, with cap off, reaching zone 3 heart rate

3-minute cool down (stand, sit, and cold shower) to reach zone 2 heart rate

*Interval 2*

5-minutes, lying down, maintaining zone 2-3 heart rate

1-minute, sitting up, reach zone 3-4 heart rate

Finish with a 5-minute cool shower

### Intermediate level

Sauna training cultivates resilience through gradual exposure. By incrementally increasing heat stress, you prompt your body's adaptive responses, harnessing the benefits of hormesis. As you increase your capacity to tolerate heat, you will advance in your practice. See a sample intermediate routine below.

*Intermediate routine*

Two intervals for a total of 35 minutes on the top shelf of a 185° sauna

*Interval 1*

8-minute minutes sitting up, warming up to open capillaries, achieving profuse sweating, and reaching zone 2 heart rate

10-minutes lying down, maintaining zone 2-3 heart rate

2 minutes sitting up, with cap off, reaching zone 3-4 heart rate

4-5 minute cool down (stand, sit, and cold shower) to reach zone 2 heart rate

*Interval 2*

8-minutes, lying down, maintaining zone 2-3 heart rate

2-minutes, sitting up, reaching zone 3-4 heart rate

Finish with a 5-minute cool shower

### Advanced level

Those in good cardiovascular fitness who are accustomed to exercising in zones 4 or 5 can tolerate more heat stress. A more demanding workout of A-B-C-D-B-C-D-B-C-D-A structure might be possible for those in top cardiovascular fitness. However, while cardiac output might not be a problem for those new to the sauna, weak capillary density might inhibit the body's ability to handle extended periods in high temperatures. Over time, with sustained exposure, the density of the capillaries in the skin will increase, allowing for more extended periods of exposure. See the sample advanced routine below.

*Advanced routine*

Three intervals for a total of 90 minutes on the top shelf of a 185° sauna

*Interval 1*

20-minute warm-up, sitting up, with a sauna cap on, to recruit capillaries, achieve profuse sweating, achieve zone 2 heart rate

20-minute lie down with heart rate between zones 2-3

5 minutes (sit up with sauna cap off) achieve zone 4-5 heart rate

4-5 minute cool down (stand, sit, and cold shower) to achieve zone 1-2 heart rate

*Interval 2*

15 minutes lying down, heart rate in zone 3

5 minutes, sitting up, achieving heart rate of zone 4

4-5 minute cool down (stand, sit, and cold shower) to achieve zone 1-2 heart rate

*Interval 3*

15 minutes lying down, heart rate in zone 3

5 minutes sitting up, achieving zone 4 heart rate

Finish with a 5-minute cool shower

**Record Your Progress**

Regardless of where you begin, try to record your progress. Keep track of the number of sessions you practice each week, the sauna temperature, the length of each session, the interval structure (the length of each interval and the physical positioning of your body), and the heart rate patterns within each interval.

You might also want to track other factors, like resting heart rate, blood pressure, blood glucose levels, sleep quality, and number of hours of sleep.

Tracking your body's growing capacity for heat tolerance and adaptation over time will provide competence feedback that will help you stay motivated as you see progress. Over time, you'll become an expert conductor of the beating of your heart.

**Adjust Your Goals to Achieve Your Aims**

Your fitness goals will determine your workout frequency, length, and structure. If you're beginning, you might decide to limit your initial sessions to short, 8-10 minute intervals to allow your body to adjust to the heat and to get in touch with the music of your heart. If you intend to use sauna practice to maintain cardiovascular fitness, you might choose a 30-40-minute workout a few times a week to maintain cardiovascular fitness. To correct bodily dysregulation while improving cardiovascular fitness, you might aim for a 50 to 60-minute daily workout. Or, if you're like me, you might aim for a 90-minute daily workout to correct bodily dysregulation, improve cardiovascular fitness, and practice mindfulness meditation (topics for discussion in the next section of the book). Once your body has adapted to extended periods of heat stress, you can use the sauna to fight viruses and infections. I've used three-hour sessions to resolve symptoms of lower urinary tract infection and two-hour sessions to resolve symptoms of strep throat. A typical 90-minute session relieves symptoms of a hangover.

As with any new training regimen, individuals should consult a healthcare professional before starting heat therapy. Certain health conditions, medications, and age-related changes in thermoregulation may affect an individual's tolerance to heat exposure. A healthcare provider can assess the individual's suitability for heat therapy and provide personalized guidance to ensure safety and effectiveness.

### What to Expect from Training: A 30-day Guide

The body's adaptation to heat exposure, often called heat acclimatization, can vary depending on the individual and the conditions, such as temperature and length of exposure. Generally, the process can be broken down into several stages. Here is what you can expect in your first month of sauna practice:

#### Days 1-5: Initial adaptation

*Increased plasma volume:* Your body will start increasing blood plasma volume, aiding cardiovascular stability and a more consistent blood flow rate.

*Reduced heart rate and core temperature:* You may notice a lower resting heart rate and a slight reduction in core body temperature during sauna sessions.

*Increased sweat rate:* Expect to sweat more as your body begins to adapt and improve cooling efficiency.

*Stress relief:* The heat will help reduce stress levels, promoting relaxation and well-being.

#### Days 6-10: Intermediate adaptation

*Improved sweat distribution:* Sweating will become more evenly distributed, enhancing cooling efficiency.

*Decreased electrolyte loss:* Your body will start conserving electrolytes (like sodium), reducing the risk of dehydration and heat cramps.

*Enhanced blood flow to skin:* Blood flow to your skin will increase, aiding in heat dissipation.

*Better sleep:* Regular sauna use can improve sleep quality, helping you fall asleep faster and enjoy deeper rest.

**Days 11-20: Advanced Adaptation**

Stabilized sweat rate: Your sweat rate will stabilize at an optimal level, enhancing your body's cooling ability.

*Optimized thermoregulation:* Your body's ability to regulate temperature will improve, making you more comfortable and efficient in the sauna.

*Continued stress reduction:* Persistent use will further decrease stress, leaving you feeling more relaxed and refreshed.

*Enhanced sleep:* Consistent heat therapy can significantly improve sleep patterns, providing more restful and restorative sleep.

**Days 21-30: Full Adaptation and Maintenance**

*Enhanced performance:* With full adaptation, you'll notice better performance and comfort during your sauna sessions.

*Maintenance:* To maintain these benefits, ensure regular sauna use. Lack of exposure for a week may lead to the beginning of adaptation loss, with complete loss possible within a few weeks of non-use.

*Ongoing stress management:* Regular sauna sessions will continue to help manage and reduce stress effectively.

*Sustained sleep quality:* Keeping up with your sauna routine will help improve sleep quality and overall well-being.

**Training in Hot Weather Conditions**

It's essential to adjust training routines in unusually hot weather conditions when the body faces a dual challenge of constant heat exposure and the physical demands of training. This combination significantly taxes the body's thermoregulatory systems, making it harder to maintain typical performance and recovery levels.

The situation is further exacerbated in locations where access to cold water is limited when even groundwater becomes tepid due to high ambient temperatures. Without access to cold water to cool down efficiently, the body struggles to dissipate heat accumulated from the environment and exercise-induced metabolic processes. As a result, the capacity for rigorous training diminishes.

The compromised ability to cool down not only limits performance during training sessions and hampers recovery between workouts, but it can also potentially lead to increased fatigue, decreased adaptation, and a higher risk of heat-related illnesses.

### *My hot-weather workout adjustments*

In extremely hot weather conditions, I modify my training. Since I take advantage of the summer months to condition my body to heat and don't use air conditioning, constant exposure to heat leads to continuous sweating and other normal physiological responses to heat. On days when temperatures linger in the high 80s to low 90s, pre-existing fatigue and dehydration significantly reduce my stamina in the sauna, making it difficult to maintain the intensity of workouts in cooler conditions. Also, I don't have access to cold water to cool my body due to higher groundwater temperatures. Tepid water doesn't provide the same degree of heat dissipation, leaving my body struggling to lower its core temperature after exertion.

To adapt to these conditions, I listen to my body, and I adjust my workout routine accordingly. I maintain a light-to-vigorous level of exercise intensity (between zones 2-3), shorten my time in the sauna, and take longer breaks. On sweltering days when I've been exposed to heat all day, my intervals are typically broken into one 30-minute interval followed by four 15-minute intervals, including five-minute breaks to bring down my heart rate.

### Conclusion

In conclusion, sauna training has emerged as a promising approach to promoting cardiovascular health and combating various diseases and bodily dysfunctions. Inducing heat stress, sauna exposure triggers a cascade of physiological responses, including increased heart rate and heat shock protein (HSP) expression. These adaptations have been shown to confer protective effects on the body, enhancing its resilience against oxidative stress, inflammation, and protein misfolding. Regular sauna sessions can potentially reverse and halt the progression of certain diseases. While further research is needed to elucidate the mechanisms and optimize the protocols fully, the training approach presented in this chapter highlights the potential of the sauna as a complementary therapy for a wide range of health conditions.

It's important to note that while the capacity to tolerate heat is in all of us, it's only realized through practice. Prolonged sauna practice is like an endurance sport—you must train your body to play the game. Once you can tolerate prolonged periods of intense heat, you will have given yourself the most powerful weapon in an arsenal of self-care that can halt and reverse disease, slow aging, fight infection, enhance sleep, and strengthen all of the body's systems. Such a profound cause warrants your devoted commitment.

# 17. ALLIED PRACTICES TO ENHANCE YOUR SAUNA JOURNEY

While regular sauna use offers numerous health benefits on its own, combining it with complementary practices can significantly amplify its positive effects on overall well-being. This chapter explores several allied practices that work synergistically with sauna bathing to optimize health and longevity.

**Diet**

The relationship between diet and sauna use is often overlooked, but it can significantly impact the effectiveness and comfort of sauna sessions. Below are suggested guidelines for a diet that works synergistically with sauna practice to enhance health.

Avoid over nutrition

Overnutrition is the excessive consumption of nutrients and calories beyond the body's requirements for normal functioning. This imbalance can lead to various health problems, including obesity, type 2 diabetes, cardiovascular diseases, and certain cancers. It typically results from overconsumption of calorie-dense foods, particularly those high in fats and sugars, and insufficient physical activity.

Researchers have shown that excessive nutrition disrupts cellular signaling, causing brown fat cells to lose their surrounding blood vessels (Shimizu et al., 2014). Cells deprived of oxygen lead to a loss of mitochondria, the cell's powerhouses. Consequently, these brown fat cells can't burn fatty acids and generate heat. This breakdown in brown fat function can significantly impact metabolic health, potentially contributing to the development of conditions like diabetes and cardiovascular disease. The findings highlight the intricate relationship between nutrition, cellular function, and overall metabolic health.

Our evolutionary ancestors likely had irregular caloric intake, with periods of abundance alternating with periods of scarcity. "If we go back to when humans were hunter-gatherers, days could pass between when they could eat, so it was a survival advantage to be able to store excess energy in white fat cells," said Kenneth Walsh, PhD, director of the Whitaker Cardiovascular Institute at Boston University School of Medicine (BUSM) and the study's senior author. Walsh continues, "What served us so well as primitive organisms are now hurting us because we have a continuous food supply and are accumulating too many white fat cells."

### Consume adequate protein

The human body relies on high protein intake from our evolutionary past as *hypercarnivores*, meaning that more than 70% of the diet was consumed from animal sources (Ben-Dor, Sirtoli & Barkai, 2021). Over millions of years, this diet shaped our anatomy and physiology, explaining why protein remains crucial for optimal bodily function, even in modern, diverse diets.

While humans are adaptable omnivores and can thrive on various diets, our long history of meat consumption has left a lasting imprint on our nutritional requirements. Protein is vital in enzyme and hormone production, immune function, and metabolic regulation. Animal proteins, in particular, provide essential amino acids in ideal proportions for human needs. Consuming adequate protein is vital for cardio endurance training, especially when combined with sauna use, as it supports muscle repair and growth. During endurance activities, muscles experience stress and microtears that require protein for effective recovery and strengthening. Additionally, protein helps sustain energy levels by stabilizing blood sugar and providing an alternative energy source when glycogen stores are depleted. It also aids in maintaining proper fluid balance, which is crucial for hydration, especially when sweating heavily in a sauna. Thus, ensuring sufficient protein intake optimizes performance, recovery, and overall endurance.

### Adopt a low-sugar diet

Maintaining a low-sugar diet can be a valuable allied practice that enhances the overall sauna experience and supports general well-being. High sugar intake can lead to several physiological changes that affect how the body responds to heat, potentially making sauna sessions less comfortable and effective.

By adopting a low-sugar diet, you can maintain proper hydration, as high blood sugar can lead to increased urination and dehydration; ensure optimal blood vessel function, allowing for better heat dissipation; minimize the metabolic heat generated by digesting large, sugary meals; and support long-term health and reduce the risk of chronic conditions like diabetes, obesity, and heart disease.

To maintain a low-sugar diet, follow these guidelines:

- Choose whole, unprocessed foods like fruits, vegetables, lean proteins, and whole grains, which naturally contain less added sugar.
- Read labels when buying packaged foods, as sugar can be disguised as fructose, dextrose, or corn syrup.
- Limit sugary drinks, a significant source of added sugars in many diets. Replacing sodas, sweetened teas, and fruit juices with water, unsweetened tea, or infused water can significantly reduce sugar intake. This switch particularly benefits sauna users, as these healthier options support hydration.
- Be mindful of portion sizes. Even healthy foods can contribute to excessive sugar consumption if eaten in large quantities. Be aware of serving sizes, especially for foods like fruits that, while nutritious, still contain natural sugars.
- Plan sauna sessions accordingly, avoiding large meals or sugary foods immediately before sessions, which leads to metabolic heat production. This additional internal heat can make sauna sessions feel more uncomfortable and

potentially reduce the body's ability to tolerate the sauna's heat.

Incorporating these low-sugar dietary practices alongside regular sauna use can create a synergistic approach to health and wellness. This combination can enhance the benefits of sauna therapy while supporting overall physiological balance and long-term health.

### Practice fasting

Humans have significantly larger body fat reserves than primates, highlighting our evolutionary adaptation to fasting. This adaptation allowed early humans to endure extended periods of fasting of several weeks, helping our ancestors cope with the unpredictable nature of hunting large prey and enabling survival when successful hunts were infrequent (Ben-Dor, Sirtoli & Barkai, 2021). The practice of fasting recreates the metabolic conditions our ancestors frequently experienced.

Fasting helps recreate hormetic stress that primes the body to operate in a fat-burning, ketogenic state of metabolism. This metabolic shift has been shown to facilitate greater heat shock protein production in response to the sauna's heat stress. More abundant heat shock proteins mean enhanced protection against cellular damage and more efficient rehabilitation of tissues. By strategically timing periods without food intake around your sauna sessions, you can activate additional pathways of cellular rejuvenation and repair and derive more therapeutic value from sauna bathing.

Fasting practices vary widely, from daily time-restricted feeding to extended multi-day fasts. Common approaches include intermittent fasting methods like the 16/8 protocol (16 hours fasting, 8 hours eating), the 5:2 diet (five normal days, two low-calorie days), and alternate-day fasting. Longer fasts of 24 to 72 hours are typically done less frequently.

Consider incorporating fasting periods of 16-24 hours before sauna sessions on a routine basis. This pre-sauna fasted state helps deplete glycogen stores and initiate the breakdown of fatty acids for energy. The sauna's thermogenic effects can then further accelerate this fat-burning mode.

Post-sauna fasting periods extending calorie restriction for a few more hours also appear to amplify many of the sauna's biochemical benefits, such as:

- Increased heat shock protein levels
- Promoted autophagy (recycling of damaged cell components)
- Activated anti-inflammatory pathways
- Enhanced insulin sensitivity
- Boosted human growth hormone production

Strategic energy deprivation can be a powerful combined stress that amplifies the rejuvenating effects of sauna bathing at a cellular level. But it's important to experiment cautiously with fasting protocols. Generally, it's advised to start with shorter fasts, stay hydrated, break your fasts gently, listen to your body, and adjust accordingly. Fasting isn't suitable for everyone, and individual responses can vary. It's advisable to consult a healthcare professional before beginning any fasting regimen, especially for extended periods.

*Fast with caution*

Evolutionary biology suggests that pre-agricultural humans fasted regularly due to inconsistent food availability. Their low-carbohydrate diets allowed for metabolic flexibility between glucose and fat-derived ketones. Modern diets, rich in carbohydrates, have altered our metabolic adaptations, potentially complicating the effects of fasting.

Recent research presented at the 2024 American Heart Association conference raises concerns about time-restricted eating. A study of over 20,000 U.S. adults over 8 years found that those following an 8-hour eating window had a 91% higher risk of cardiovascular mortality compared to those with 12- to 16-hour eating periods. This finding is particularly relevant for individuals with pre-existing heart conditions or cancer.

Given these insights, it's advisable to approach fasting cautiously, considering it as one potential tool within a broader health strategy rather than a universal solution.

*My fasting practice*

I come from a family of overeaters who relied on fasting to manage our weight. As a teenager, I experimented with various fasting methods. My father, a physician, once had us try a week-long ketosis fast using a thick, unpleasant protein syrup. Later, I adopted monthly week-long fasts with meal replacement drinks. My sister and I practiced intermittent fasting in college, often not eating after 5:00 p.m. This habit has stuck with me into adulthood. Now, I typically practice intermittent fasting, usually delaying my first meal until the afternoon.

I recently did a five-day zero-calorie fast as a strategy to lose weight after a stressful year and an extra 15 pounds on the scale. I was inspired by the research of Dr. Ian Lake (2021), who, along with seven other subjects, ran one marathon every day for five days while fasting to show that ketosis was safe for type 1 diabetics. The subjects lost an average of seven pounds without losing significant muscle. I modified Lake's experiment. I did a five-day zero-calorie fast, but instead of running a marathon each day, I spent three hours in the sauna daily (two 90-minute sessions) to achieve a similar level of cardiac output. I also took an appetite suppressant on the first day called Zepbound to avoid discomfort. My weight was 179 when I weighed myself the first day on the scale at my gym. I weighed myself on a smart scale the second through fifth days. I lost a total of 14 pounds over the five-day fast; Figure 17-1 shows my weight from days two through five. My current weight is 169. To maintain weight, I consume a very low-sugar, mostly carnivore diet. And to lose more weight, I'll do a multiple-day fast again and again until I achieve my ideal weight.

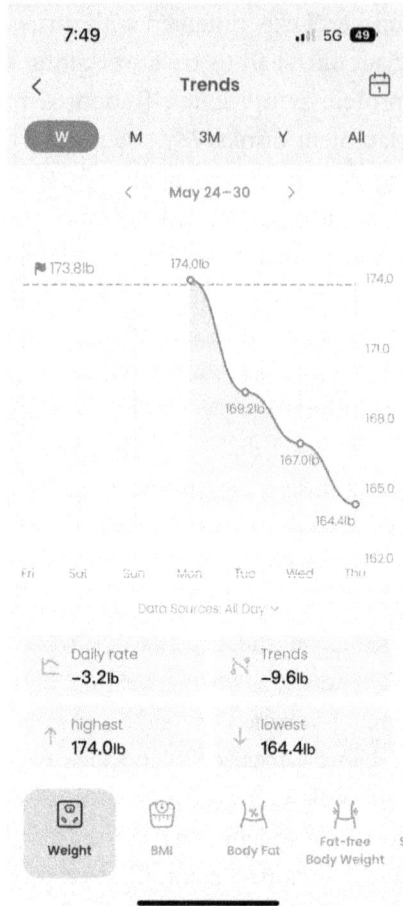

*Figure 17-1: Weight-loss trends from Days 2-5 of a five-day fast.*

### Breathwork

Breathwork is a powerful practice that harnesses the potential of controlled breathing to enhance physical, mental, and emotional well-being. This ancient technique, found in various cultures and traditions, has gained renewed interest in modern wellness circles. By consciously altering breathing patterns, practitioners can activate the body's relaxation response, reduce stress, improve focus, and boost energy levels. Breathwork can also help regulate the autonomic nervous system, potentially alleviating symptoms of anxiety and depression. From simple deep breathing exercises to more complex breathwork practices, this versatile tool offers a range of benefits accessible to people of all ages and fitness levels, making it a valuable addition to any wellness routine.

Certain breathing techniques involve controlled hyperventilation followed by breath retention. This process can lead to a temporary increase in blood pH levels (respiratory alkalosis) and a decrease in blood $CO_2$ levels. The combination of heat stress from the sauna and the altered blood chemistry from breathwork work synergistically to enhance the expression of heat shock proteins (HSPs). The low $CO_2$ levels in the blood caused by hyperventilation can simulate a state of hypoxia (low oxygen), another stressor that can trigger HSP production. As discussed, increased HSP expression can help improve the body's resilience to various stressors, including oxidative stress, inflammation, and toxins, contributing to better overall health and longevity.

When practicing breathwork in the intense heat of a sauna, it's crucial to exercise caution: listen to your body, exit immediately if you feel dizzy or lightheaded, and stay well-hydrated before, during, and after your session to prevent dehydration and potential heat-related illnesses. Breathwork is discussed in greater detail in the chapter, *Sauna Prana*.

I incorporate a breathwork exercise into the first five minutes of my sauna session. Here's a paragraph describing your sauna breathwork routine:

### My breathwork routine

During the first five minutes of my sauna session, I engage in a structured breathwork routine consisting of three intervals. I begin by taking slow, deep breaths in through my nose and exhaling forcefully through my mouth. The first interval involves 10 such breaths, followed by holding my breath for a slow count to 10 after the final exhale. In the second interval, I increase to 20 breaths, again holding my breath for 20 seconds at the end. The final interval consists of 30 breaths, culminating in an extended breath hold. After completing these breathing exercises, I transition into a meditative state, focusing on listening to my intuition for the remainder of my sauna session. This practice combines controlled breathing techniques with meditation, potentially enhancing the benefits of my sauna experience.

## Exercise Routines to Enhance Physical Fitness

Incorporating an exercise regimen into your routine can complement your sauna practice by enhancing overall health and fitness.

### Goals

Exercise goals provide direction, motivation, and a clear framework for progress. They help you stay focused, measure your achievements, and maintain consistency in your fitness journey, ultimately leading to achieving your aims.

First, determine your fitness goals. Good fitness goals are specific, measurable, achievable, relevant, and time-bound (SMART). They can encompass various aspects of physical health and well-being, including cardiovascular endurance (e.g., completing a 5K run), strength training (increasing weight lifted in specific exercises), flexibility and mobility (improving range of motion), body composition (reducing body fat percentage or gaining lean muscle), and functional fitness (enhancing balance and core strength).

Health-related goals like lowering blood pressure or improving insulin sensitivity can also be valuable. Additionally, consistency goals such as establishing a regular exercise routine are essential for long-term success. It's crucial to set both short-term and long-term goals, regularly reassess progress, and adjust as needed. Remember to consult healthcare professionals or certified fitness instructors when setting fitness goals, especially if you have pre-existing health conditions.

### Types of exercise

Next, plan a routine to enable you to achieve your goals. Consider incorporating any of these activities:

#### Cardiovascular exercise

Activities like running, cycling, swimming, or using cardio machines engage multiple muscle groups to tax the cardiovascular system significantly, promoting enhanced heart function and resilience. These exercises increase heart rate, strengthen the heart muscle, improve circulation, and boost overall endurance. Over time, consistent cardio training can lead to better oxygen delivery to tissues, improved metabolic efficiency, and reduced risk of cardiovascular diseases.

#### Strength training

Weight lifting can significantly enhance muscle mass and bone density, supporting overall physical strength and reducing osteoporosis risk. It also boosts metabolism by increasing the amount of lean muscle tissue, which burns more calories at rest. Additionally, weight lifting improves insulin sensitivity, aiding in better blood sugar regulation and reducing the risk of type 2 diabetes. Furthermore, it can enhance cardiovascular health by lowering blood pressure, improving circulation, and promoting heart health through increased physical activity.

*Flexibility and mobility workouts*

Stretching, yoga, or Pilates can significantly enhance flexibility by lengthening muscles and increasing the range of motion in joints. These activities also improve balance by strengthening core muscles and promoting body awareness, which helps prevent falls and injuries. Additionally, they enhance joint mobility by maintaining and increasing the fluidity and health of the connective tissues and lubricating the joints, leading to greater ease of movement and reduced stiffness. Regular practice of these disciplines contributes to better posture, reduced muscle tension, and overall physical and mental well-being.

### Intensity and progression

When combining exercise training with sauna use, following a few key guidelines to maximize benefits and prevent adverse effects is essential.

First, adhere to the principle of progressive overload by gradually increasing the intensity and difficulty of your workouts. This approach ensures continuous improvement in strength, endurance, and overall fitness.

Additionally, it is crucial to allow adequate recovery time between intense exercise sessions and sauna use to prevent overtraining and reduce the risk of injury. Using the sauna post-workout can significantly enhance recovery by promoting muscle relaxation and reducing inflammation.

Staying well-hydrated throughout the process is vital, as both exercise and sauna sessions can lead to significant fluid loss. Drinking plenty of water before, during, and after workouts and sauna sessions will help maintain optimal hydration levels, support recovery, and ensure your fitness regimen's safety and effectiveness.

### Sleep Hygiene

Quality sleep is crucial for overall health and can significantly enhance the benefits of your sauna practice. Sleep is vital to overall health, well-being, and physical and mental restoration. Quality sleep helps regulate hormones, supports immune function, and facilitates cellular repair processes. It's essential for cognitive functions such as memory consolidation, learning, and emotional regulation. Consistent, restful sleep can improve mood, increase productivity, and reduce the risk of various health issues, including obesity, cardiovascular disease, and mental health disorders. Establishing a regular sleep schedule, creating a conducive sleep environment, and incorporating relaxation techniques can all contribute to better sleep quality. Individuals can optimize their overall well-being and quality of life by prioritizing sleep as part of a holistic approach to health, alongside practices like sauna use, proper nutrition, and exercise.

Good sleep hygiene includes:

- Maintaining a consistent sleep schedule involves going to bed and waking up at the same time every day, which helps regulate your body's internal clock and can improve the quality of your sleep. Creating an optimal sleep environment means ensuring your bedroom is cool, quiet, and dark, which can enhance your ability to fall and stay asleep.
- Limiting exposure to screens before bedtime is crucial because the blue light emitted from phones, tablets, and computers can interfere with the production of melatonin, a hormone that regulates sleep.
- Avoiding stimulants such as caffeine and heavy meals close to bedtime can prevent disruptions to your sleep by reducing the likelihood of indigestion or heightened alertness.
- Practicing relaxation techniques, such as deep breathing, meditation, or gentle stretching, can calm your mind and body, making it easier to transition into a restful sleep.

Sauna use can contribute to better sleep by promoting relaxation and helping to regulate your body's internal clock. Consider incorporating sauna sessions into your evening routine to help prepare your body for restful sleep.

**Supplementation**

While a balanced diet should be the primary source of nutrients, certain supplements may help enhance the effects of sauna use by supporting the body's natural detoxification processes and promoting overall health. However, it is important to note that deficiencies in micronutrients vary by individual depending on health status, dietary habits, and the condition of the microbiome. It is important to consult with a healthcare professional before starting any new supplement regimen.

***Electrolytes***

Sweating during sauna sessions can lead to losing essential electrolytes like sodium, potassium, and magnesium. Replenishing these electrolytes through supplements can help maintain proper hydration and body functions.

***Micronutrients***

Micronutrients are essential vitamins and minerals required in small amounts for proper growth, development, and physiological functioning.

*Micronutrients and the microbiome*

The demand for micronutrients is closely related to the quality of the microbiome. The microbiome is the collection of all the microorganisms, including bacteria, fungi, viruses, and their genes, that live in and on the human body, playing a crucial role in health and disease.

A healthy microbiome enhances the absorption of essential micronutrients like B vitamins, vitamin K, iron, and magnesium. In contrast, a poor-quality microbiome can hinder this process, leading to deficiencies even with an adequate diet. Certain gut bacteria can synthesize essential vitamins, contributing to overall health, but an imbalanced microbiome can reduce this natural synthesis.

The microbiome also plays a crucial role in regulating the immune system. A compromised microbiome can increase the body's demand for nutrients like vitamins A, C, D, and zinc to maintain immune balance.

Additionally, a healthy microbiome helps maintain gut integrity and reduces inflammation, which can otherwise increase the need for antioxidants and anti-inflammatory nutrients. The microbiome influences metabolic processes, affecting how the body processes carbohydrates and fats, with micronutrients like chromium and B vitamins essential for metabolic health. Moreover, the gut-brain axis highlights the connection between gut health and mental well-being, with micronutrients such as magnesium, vitamin D, and omega-3 fatty acids playing a role in brain health. Therefore, maintaining a diverse and balanced gut microbiota through a diet rich in fiber, probiotics, prebiotics, and adequate micronutrient intake is crucial for overall health and well-being.

*Micronutrient deficiencies*

Micronutrient deficiencies are the most common type of nutritional deficiency and occur due to inadequate intake of essential micronutrients necessary for optimal health (Kiani et al., 2022). Key micronutrients include iron, iodine, calcium, zinc, magnesium, fluoride, and vitamins A, B6, B12, C, D, E, and K. A list of micronutrients and their functions appears below. Dietary supplementation is a major strategy for managing these deficiencies, as it helps increase the intake of underconsumed nutrients and bridges nutritional gaps in the population (IBID).

- Iron: Essential for the formation of hemoglobin, which carries oxygen in the blood.
- Iodine: Necessary for the production of thyroid hormones, which regulate metabolism.
- Calcium: Vital for the development and maintenance of strong bones and teeth and plays a role in muscle function, nerve signaling, and blood clotting.
- Zinc: Important for immune function, wound healing, DNA synthesis, and cell division.
- Magnesium: Involved in over 300 biochemical reactions in the body, including muscle and nerve function, blood glucose control, and protein synthesis.
- Fluoride: Helps prevent dental cavities by making teeth more resistant to acid attacks from plaque bacteria and sugars in the mouth. Some research suggests ingestion
- Folate (Vitamin B9): Essential for DNA synthesis and repair, red

blood cell formation, preventing neural tube defects in pregnancy, breaking down homocysteine for heart health, and supporting mental and immune function.

• Vitamin A: This antioxidant supports the immune system and helps protect cells from oxidative stress. It also aids in producing glutathione, a crucial antioxidant for detoxification. It is crucial for vision and skin health. Research suggests that higher vitamin C needs result from higher carbohydrate consumption and higher blood glucose levels in Western populations, and very low carbohydrate diets high in animal foods can decrease the body's need for vitamin C (Ben-Dor, Sirtoli & Barkai, 2021).

• Vitamin B6: Important for brain development and function and helps the body convert food into energy.

• Vitamin B12: Essential for nerve tissue health, brain function, and the production of red blood cells.

• Vitamin C: Necessary for the growth, development, and repair of all body tissues, and is involved in many body functions, including the absorption of iron, the immune system, wound healing, and the mainte-nance of cartilage, bones, and teeth.

• Vitamin D: Important for the absorption of calcium and phos-phorus, which are needed to maintain healthy bones and teeth. Essential for immune function and mental well-being. Deficiency can lead to bone disorders, weakened immune response, and mood disorders.

• Vitamin E: Acts as an antioxidant, helping to protect cells from the damage caused by free radicals.

• Vitamin K: Essential for blood clotting and helps maintain bone health.

• Omega-3 Fatty Acids: These healthy fats, found in fish oil supple-ments, support cardiovascular health, reduce inflammation, and promote overall well-being.

*Micronutrients and carnivore diet*

Eating a diet high in animal sources might provide natural nutrients, thus reducing the need for supplementation. Research suggests that a diet high in animal-sourced foods provides essential nutrients in higher quantities in their most effective forms that plants can't, including vitamin A (retinol), vitamin K2, vitamin B9 (folate), vitamin B12, vitamin B6, vitamin D, iron, and omega-3 fatty acids (EPA and DHA) (Ben-Dor, Sirtoli & Barkai, 2021).

**Co-enzyme NAD+**

NAD+ (nicotinamide adenine dinucleotide) is a crucial molecule in energy metabolism and cellular functions, which may decline with age. Advocates claim that boosting NAD+ levels can improve cellular energy production, support DNA repair, enhance cognitive function, enhance metabolic health, and promote healthy aging (see Sinclaire & LaPlante, 2019).

While you could theoretically take NAD+ directly, it isn't the most effective way to increase NAD+ levels in the body. NAD+ is a large molecule that may not be efficiently absorbed orally. Instead, taking NAD+ precursors like nicotinamide riboside (NR) or nicotinamide mononucleotide (NMN) is more effective. These precursors are smaller molecules that the body can absorb and convert into NAD+. This method ensures better bioavailability and efficacy, helping to raise NAD+ levels more reliably. Additionally, NAD+ supplements and their precursors are more stable and easier to formulate, making them a practical choice for supplementation.

Especially relevant to sauna practice and the role of the circulatory system in regulating body temperature, some research suggests that NMN may also promote angiogenesis, the formation of new blood vessels. This effect could occur through various mechanisms, such as improving vascular health, activating SIRT1 (a protein involved in angiogenesis), enhancing endothelial function, and providing the cellular energy necessary for new vessel formation.

While some studies suggest potential benefits, more research is needed to fully understand the efficacy and long-term safety of NAD+ supplementation. As with any supplement, it is advisable to consult with a healthcare professional before starting NAD+ supplements.

**General Heat Hacks: Alternative Ways to Stimulate Heat Adaptation**

While regular sauna use offers potent health benefits, there are numerous other ways to expose your body to heat and stimulate adaptive responses. These *heat hacks* can complement your sauna practice or serve as alternatives when a sauna isn't available:

### Embrace natural heat

During warmer months, limit air conditioning use. Allow your body to acclimate to higher temperatures naturally, which can improve heat tolerance and stimulate physiological adaptations.

### Hot car therapy

A car parked in the sun on a hot day can feel like a sauna inside. You can take advantage of the opportunity by sitting in your car to trigger the heat stress response and mimic a sauna session.

### Hot baths

Immerse yourself in a hot bath (around 104°F/40°C) for 20-30 minutes. This can induce similar physiological responses to sauna bathing, including increased heart rate and blood flow.

### Exercise in warm environments

Engage in light to moderate exercise in warmer settings, either outdoors or in a heated room. This combines the benefits of exercise with heat exposure. Try hot yoga or pilates, combining stretching and strength exercises with heat exposure.

### Ambient heat exposure

Spend time outdoors during peak sun hours, but do so safely. Seek partial shade or use a broad-spectrum sunscreen to shield your skin from UV radiation while benefiting from the ambient heat.

These heat hacks can help you harness some of the benefits of heat exposure when a traditional sauna isn't available, complementing your overall heat therapy regimen. But remember, while these methods can offer benefits, they should be approached gradually and cautiously, especially if you have pre-existing health conditions. Always stay hydrated and listen to your body's signals.

### Conclusion

Incorporating these allied practices into your routine alongside regular sauna use can create a holistic approach to health and wellness. Remember to listen to your body, start gradually, and consult with healthcare professionals when necessary. As you combine these practices, you may find that the synergistic effects lead to even more significant improvements in your overall well-being and quality of life.

# PART FOUR
# SAUNA NIRVANA

Nirvana is a state of spiritual enlightenment characterized by profound peace, happiness, insight into reality's true nature, and freedom from suffering. It's the ultimate goal of spiritual practice.

Beyond physical benefits, the real magic of sauna practice lies in its power to create mental clarity, emotional balance, and spiritual connection.

My sauna journey began with a focus on physical fitness, but evolved into a holistic, spiritually oriented practice that enabled me to cultivate balance, inner peace, and well-being amidst health challenges.

As you develop your practice, you may become more attuned to your body's needs, resilient to stress, and connected to your authentic self.

This section explores how consistent, prolonged sauna practice can instill peace, contentment, and joy—the core of well-being. It explores concepts and practices that can support your journey towards sauna nirvana, such as meditation, breathwork, and social connection. By aligning your sauna sessions with the pursuit of nirvana, you can create a sacred space for personal discovery and transformation, tap into your inherent wisdom and clarity, and unlock the sauna's vast potential for personal growth.

# 18. Sauna Spirituality

Ancient wisdom traditions like yoga and meditation view physical training as a pathway to spiritual enlightenment and self-realization rather than an end in itself. The body is prepared for higher consciousness through various techniques in these practices. Yoga uses physical postures to strengthen the body and balance energy, fostering inner stillness and self-awareness. Meditation employs physical discipline to build mental clarity and insight, using the body as a foundation for more profound spiritual work. Physical training is a means to a higher end.

In contrast, Western approaches to physical training are often employed to achieve external goals. Sports training focuses on performance, skill development, and achieving victory in competition. Western fitness culture pursues health benefits, aesthetic improvements, and embraces the "no pain, no gain" mentality.

My journey with sauna practice began with a Western mindset, primarily seeking improved cardiovascular performance. However, it evolved into a fusion of physical benefits and spiritual growth, supporting a more holistic approach to well-being and personal development. The sauna became a sacred space for heightened awareness and introspection, where I learned to embrace physical discomfort as a portal to profound calm and clarity.

As I committed to daily practice, I found myself able to access deeper aspects of my being. Over time, symptoms of anxiety and depression gradually diminished. A growing sense of self-authenticity enabled me to confront and cope with long-standing fears, doubts, and limiting beliefs. As my practice deepened, it evolved to support a meditative state that fostered a sense of interconnectedness with the universe—a state that I came to call "sauna nirvana."

While the physical benefits of sauna therapy remain significant, the spiritual dimension has become the primary motivation for my daily practice—a sacred daily ritual and a pilgrimage into the depths of my being. This chapter explores dimensions of sauna spirituality so that you, too, can begin your journey toward nirvana.

**Sauna Zen: The Practice of Heat-induced Conscious Awareness**

Zen, a branch of Buddhism that originated in China, emphasizes direct insight into the nature of consciousness through meditation and direct pointing to the mind. It stresses the importance of direct, non-conceptual awareness of the present moment. This bare attention reveals the fluid, impermanent nature of conscious experience and the lack of a fixed, independent self.

Through practices like *shikantaza* ("just sitting"), Zen practitioners aim to cut through the illusions of the discursive mind and awaken to the non-dual nature of reality, where subject and object, mind and world, aren't fundamentally separate. Zen points to the inherently empty, boundless nature of awareness beneath all temporary contents of consciousness. Realizing this "original mind" or "Buddha-nature" is the key to liberation. Zen also recognizes the transformative potential of altered states of consciousness, as evidenced by sudden awakening experiences (satori) that can radically shift one's perception of reality. Within this unified state in which the practitioner is fully immersed in the moment, free from the distractions of the mind and the external world, the boundaries between self and other, inner and outer, begin to dissolve, giving rise to a profound sense of unity and interconnectedness.

In many ancient contemplative practices, extreme heat was sometimes used in a controlled spiritual context to induce altered states of consciousness under the guidance of experienced practitioners. In some Native American traditions like the Lakota, sweat lodge ceremonies involved prolonged exposure to steam and high heat for prayer and purification. The heat and dehydration could lead to altered consciousness. Certain ancient Mesoamerican cultures, like the Aztecs and Mayans, had purification rituals and healing practices involving sweat baths called temazcals. The enclosed stone structures generated intense heat that could cause dissociation and visions. The Scandinavian saunas are thought to have originated as a shamanic practice. The extreme heat was believed to cleanse the body and mind, allowing people to reach ecstatic trance states.

### Sauna Meditation

The sauna's heat and stillness create the perfect conditions for this kind of deep, meditative awareness, allowing access to mental clarity that can be difficult to achieve in daily life. During prolonged exposure to extreme heat, thoughts of the rational mind are too burdensome to maintain. The mind is quieted, and a unique state of consciousness emerges.

Access to this unique state occurs partly because prolonged sauna sessions can induce physiological changes that may lead to shifts in consciousness and heightened mindfulness. Here's how:

After about 15 minutes in a sauna of 180°F, the core body temperature increases by about 1.5-2.5°, leading to changes in cognitive function. Heat-induced cognitive changes in the sauna share parallels with the effects of meditation. Extended exposure to heat stress causes the body to release endorphins, natural pain-relieving and mood-enhancing chemicals. This endorphin rush can lead to euphoria, relaxation, and increased well-being, promoting a more positive and present-focused state of mind.

### *Altered brain waves*

Combining heat, relaxation, and endorphins may alter brain wave patterns. Brain waves are rhythmic patterns of electrical activity produced by neurons in the brain. These patterns can be measured using an electroencephalogram (EEG). There are five main types of brain waves, each associated with different states of consciousness and mental activity:

1. Delta waves (0.5-4 Hz):
- Slowest waves
- Associated with deep, dreamless sleep and unconsciousness
- Important for healing and regeneration

2. Theta waves (4-8 Hz):
- Linked to deep relaxation, meditation, and light sleep
- Often associated with creativity, insight, and memory recall

3. Alpha waves (8-13 Hz):
- Present during relaxed wakefulness, especially with closed eyes
- Associated with calmness, relaxation, and improved mood

4. Beta waves (13-30 Hz):
- Dominant during normal waking consciousness
- Associated with active thinking, problem-solving, and concentration

5. Gamma waves (30-100 Hz):
- Fastest brain waves
- Linked to higher cognitive functions, including perception, problem-solving, and consciousness
- Associated with peak performance states and heightened awareness

The brain produces combinations of these waves at different times, depending on our mental state and activities.

Sauna use can increase alpha and theta brain waves associated with relaxation, meditation, and creative thinking. This shift in brain activity may contribute to a more introspective and self-aware state of consciousness.

### Present-moment awareness (suppression of the Default Mode Network)

Like meditation, heat-induced cognitive changes can reduce mental chatter and increase present-moment awareness by suppressing what is known as the Default Mode Network (DMN). The DMN is a set of interconnected brain regions active during wakeful rest, such as daydreaming or mind-wandering. It primarily functions in introspection, autobiographical memory, social cognition, and future planning. The DMN is most active when the mind isn't engaged in specific tasks.

Its activity decreases during focused attention or meditation. Overactivity of the DMN has been linked to conditions like depression and anxiety.

### Sensory deprivation

The quiet, enclosed space of a sauna can create a mildly sensory-deprived environment. This reduction in external stimuli can help individuals turn their attention inward, promoting self-reflection and mindfulness. The lack of distractions allows for a more focused and present-centered experience.

### Deep breathing

The hot air in a sauna can make breathing more challenging, often leading to slower, deeper, and more rhythmic breathing patterns. This type of controlled breathing is similar to techniques used in meditation and can help calm the mind, reduce stress, and increase mindfulness.

### Mental resilience

Prolonged heat exposure is a form of physical stress that challenges the body's homeostasis. As the body adapts to this stress over time, it can build resilience and improve stress tolerance. This enhanced ability to handle physical stress may translate to better emotional and mental resilience, supporting a more stable and aware state of consciousness.

### The Effortlessness of Heat-induced Consciousness

One advantage of heat-induced altered state of consciousness is that it is relatively effortless to achieve compared to deliberate meditation, which can be challenging.

The Indian yoga guru, mystic, and author Sadhguru (n.d.) explains that many find meditation hard because they are trying to *do* it. He explains, "You cannot do meditation but you can become meditative. Meditation is a certain quality. It is not a certain act. If you cultivate your body, your mind, your energies and your emotions to a certain level of maturity, meditation will naturally happen...If you learn to keep your body absolutely still, then your mind will also become still."

### My Sauna Zen

My 90-minute daily sauna routine allows me to effortlessly meditate for up to an hour each session. The practice of regular, deep meditation has dramatically calmed my nervous system and enabled me to tame the kind of wandering thoughts that perpetuate depression and anxiety.

**A Word of Caution**

Both the experiences of meditation and heat exposure can lead to beneficial adaptations over time. However, while meditation is a deliberate practice of mental training, heat-induced cognitive changes are a physiological response to environmental stress. It's crucial to approach heat exposure cautiously, as extreme temperatures can be dangerous, unlike meditation, which is generally safe when practiced correctly.

**Conclusion**

In conclusion, the practice of Sauna Zen offers a unique fusion of ancient wisdom and modern wellness. This chapter has explored how the intense heat of the sauna can induce a state of heightened consciousness, similar to deep meditation, but with the advantage of being more effortlessly achieved. The physiological changes brought about by prolonged heat exposure—including altered brain wave patterns, endorphin release, and suppression of the Default Mode Network—create an ideal environment for introspection, mindfulness, and spiritual growth.

The sauna becomes more than just a space for physical rejuvenation; it transforms into a sacred arena for personal development and self-discovery. By embracing the discomfort of heat and using it as a gateway to deeper awareness, practitioners can access states of consciousness that foster clarity, reduce anxiety and depression, and promote a sense of interconnectedness with the universe.

This holistic approach to sauna practice, combining physical benefits with spiritual growth, offers a powerful tool for those seeking to enhance their overall well-being.

# 19. SAUNA PRANA

The concept of *prana* has its roots in ancient Indian philosophy and spirituality, dating back thousands of years. In the religious and philosophical tradition of *Vedicism*, which laid the foundation for Hinduism, prana is considered the vital life force energy that permeates all living beings and the universe itself. It is believed to be the essential substrate that sustains life, animating the body and mind and connecting the individual to the cosmic whole.

The Vedic texts, such as the Upanishads and the Bhagavad Gita, emphasize the importance of prana in maintaining health, vitality, and longevity. They describe how prana flows through a network of energy channels called *nadis*, nourishing the body and mind, and explain how imbalances in the flow of prana can lead to disease and dysfunction.

The practices of *pranayama*, or breathwork, were developed to cultivate, balance, and harness the power of prana. Through controlled breathing techniques, such as deep diaphragmatic breathing, alternate nostril breathing, and breath retention, practitioners aimed to purify the nadis, increase the flow of prana, and promote physical, mental, and spiritual well-being. These ancient breathwork practices find their modern-day equivalents in the techniques often incorporated into sauna rituals. Techniques for pranayama, or breathwork, during sauna practice will be discussed later in this chapter.

**Prana and VO2 max**

The ancient practice of harnessing prana finds remarkable parallels in the contemporary understanding of cardiovascular fitness and the role of oxygen intake in energy production and bodily rejuvenation. The modern understanding of VO2 max, or the maximum volume of oxygen the body can take in during intense physical activity, provides a scientific framework for understanding the ancient concept of prana. Just as prana is seen as the vital energy that sustains life, oxygen plays a crucial role in the body's energy production processes. By enhancing oxygen intake and utilization through sauna sessions and breathwork practices, individuals can tap into the revitalizing power of prana and support their body's natural rejuvenation processes.

In a sauna session, heat stress induces physiological responses that closely mimic the effects of pranayama. The elevated temperature causes the heart rate to increase, blood vessels to dilate, and sweat production intensifies, leading to enhanced blood circulation and improved oxygen delivery to the tissues and organs. Increased oxygen intake and utilization mirror the concept of prana as the vital energy that sustains life and promotes rejuvenation.

An increased cardiac output in the sauna means more blood is circulated through the body per minute. Since blood carries oxygen (bound to hemoglobin in red blood cells), more blood flow results in more oxygen being transported throughout the body. The primary purpose of circulating more blood is to meet the increased oxygen demands of tissues. When your heart rate goes up, it is typically a response to your body's need for more energy and oxygen. Thus, a higher heart rate, within an optimal range, can effectively increase the circulation of blood and oxygen delivery to where it is needed most. This adaptation is particularly crucial during periods of physical activity or stress when the oxygen and nutrient demands of the body are higher.

Increasing oxygen intake can significantly enhance your overall health and well-being. It boosts energy levels and cognitive function by improving ATP production, leading to better mental clarity and focus. Athletes benefit from enhanced performance and endurance due to faster oxygen delivery to muscles. A well-oxygenated body supports immune function, helping white blood cells combat pathogens more effectively. Deep breathing and increased oxygen intake also promote relaxation and stress reduction. Oxygen is crucial in detoxification, breaking down toxins for easier elimination. It accelerates healing and recovery, particularly in damaged tissues, and is often used in medical treatments. Lastly, higher oxygen intake supports cardiovascular health by improving heart function and blood circulation, benefiting the entire body.

Moreover, sauna heat exposure triggers the release of heat shock proteins, which facilitate cellular rejuvenation. The ancient understanding of prana as a force that promotes vitality and longevity can describe the effects of increased oxygen intake and HSP expression in the body.

The relaxation and stress-reducing effects of sauna bathing also parallel the ancient concept of prana. In Vedic philosophy, stress and mental agitation are seen as disruptions to the balanced flow of prana, leading to a sense of disconnection and *dis*-ease. Inducing deep relaxation, sauna sessions help alleviate stress, allowing the body to optimize its oxygen intake and energy production mechanisms and restore balance and harmony.

**Breathwork Activities**

In the intense heat of the sauna, our breath becomes a powerful ally. This section presents breathwork techniques that transform the sauna experience into a practice of mind-body integration. By harnessing the breath, the sauna becomes a space for profound physiological and psychological transformation.

*Centering Breath*

Begin by settling into the sauna and becoming aware of your breath. Take slow, deep breaths through the nose, filling your lungs completely, then exhale slowly through the mouth. Repeat for 5-10 cycles to center yourself.

*Box Breathing*

Inhale for a count of 4, hold for 4, exhale for 4, and hold empty for 4. Repeat this cycle for 5-10 rounds. This technique can help calm the mind and regulate the nervous system.

### Cooling Breath (Sitali)

Roll your tongue into a tube (or purse your lips if you can't roll your tongue). Inhale through this tube, feeling the cooling sensation. Close your mouth and exhale through your nose. This practice can help cool the body in the sauna's heat.

### Alternate Nostril Breathing

Use your thumb to close your right nostril and inhale through the left. Then close the left with your ring finger, open the right, and exhale. Inhale right, exhale left. Continue alternating for 5-10 cycles.

### Ocean Breath (Ujjayi)

Inhale deeply through your nose. On the exhale, slightly constrict the back of your throat to create a soft "ocean" sound. This breath can be both calming and energizing.

### Wim Hof Power Breathing

Sit comfortably and take 30-40 quick, deep breaths, inhaling through the nose or mouth and exhaling through the mouth. Feel your chest and belly expand. After the last exhale, hold your breath for as long as it is comfortable. When you need to breathe, take one deep breath and hold for 15 seconds.

### Breath Retention Heat Tolerance

Take 20 deep, rhythmic breaths. On the last exhale, hold your breath for as long as it is comfortable. During this hold, focus on relaxing your body and mind, accepting the sauna's heat. When you need to breathe, inhale deeply and hold for 15 seconds. Repeat 2-3 times. This exercise can help increase heat tolerance and mind-body connection.

### Use Caution

In the intense heat of a sauna, performing multiple cycles of breathwork techniques can be significantly more challenging than under normal conditions. It is crucial to approach sauna breathwork cautiously and respect one's physical limits. The sauna's high temperature already places considerable stress on the body. This physiological stress can make it more difficult to perform controlled breathing exercises, especially those involving breath retention or rapid breathing. Keep these concerns in mind:

### Dehydration risk

Rapid breathing can accelerate water loss, which is already heightened in the sauna.

### Overheating

Heat exposure and intense breathwork could lead to overheating more quickly.

### Dizziness or lightheadedness

The heat combined with altered breathing patterns might cause these symptoms more readily.

### Cardiovascular strain

The heart is already working harder in the sauna; intense breathwork could add to this strain.

### Reduced lung capacity

The hot, dry air in the sauna can make deep breathing more challenging.

Always prioritize safety and listen to your body, potentially reducing the number of cycles or the duration of breath holds to avoid overexertion in the intense heat environment. Breathwork can be physically demanding; endurance must be gradually developed through consistent practice, like any exercise. It's crucial to start slowly, listen to your body's signals, and progressively build your ability to avoid overexertion or discomfort over time. As a critical safety precaution, always leave the sauna immediately if you feel dizzy, lightheaded, or unusually uncomfortable, as these could be signs of heat exhaustion or dehydration.

By balancing the potential benefits with necessary precautions, sauna breathwork can become a transformative practice, offering a path to enhanced vitality, stress reduction, and a deeper mind-body connection.

### Conclusion

In conclusion, breathwork in the sauna offers a powerful synergy between ancient wisdom and a modern understanding of physiology. By incorporating mindful breathing techniques into sauna sessions, practitioners can potentially enhance oxygen intake, improve circulation, and boost overall health and well-being. The sauna environment amplifies the effects of breathwork, creating a unique opportunity for profound physiological and psychological transformation.

## 20. Integration, Harmony and Well-being
### Sauna as a Somatonous Practice

In the realm of wellness, few concepts are as transformative as *integration*. Integration, in psychological terms, is the process of harmoniously connecting and coordinating different aspects of the mind, brain, and relationships, leading to a more coherent, flexible, and adaptive state of being. Somatonous is a novel word that combines the Greek root, soma, meaning body, with 'nous,' meaning mind. Practice that link the body and mind can be considered *somatonous*.

A body of science that can inform how we think about somatonous practice is Interpersonal Neurobiology (IPNB). IPNB, led by Dr. Daniel J. Siegel, is a discipline that explores the interconnections between the brain, mind, and relationships (2012a, 2012b, 2018, 2020). Siegle's work has been instrumental in illuminating the processes of integration, which is a key concept in IPNB.

Siegel defines integration as the linkage of differentiated parts of a system, whether that system is the brain, the mind, or relationships. In the brain, it's coordination between different neural networks. In the mind, it's a harmonious connection between various aspects of mental processes, like thoughts, feelings, and memories. In relationships, it's when individuals maintain their unique identities while forming meaningful connections with others. Siegle asserts that well-being is the state of integration.

This chapter draws on Dr. Siegel's work to explore the sauna as an ideal space for somatonous practice.

### Integration through Three-pillar Practice

Siegel's approach to integration and well-being focuses on what he refers to as *Three-Pillar Practices*. Three Pillar Practice is a framework for cultivating well-being and integration through mindfulness achieved through *focused attention*, *open awareness*, and *kind intention*. The three pillars are described below:

#### 1. Focused attention

This pillar involves training the mind to guide and control the flow of energy and information. Selective attention, as described by Kandel (2006), functions as a filter, choosing certain stimuli for further processing by the brain. In the context of the 3-pillar practice, individuals train their selective attention, or what Siegel refers to as focal attention, to be guided, allowing experiences to be selectively brought into awareness.

Focused attention acts as a gateway to change by driving specific experiences into awareness, setting the stage for the growth of neural connections. As Siegel notes, "Where attention goes, neural firing flows and neural connection grows." This process facilitates neuroplastic growth, altering the brain's structure and function.

Focused attention *generates* specific neural firing patterns that transform temporary states into enduring traits. Siegel refers to the deliberate guidance of attention as "guiding flow." The ability to guide and regulate the flow of energy and information in the system enables you to potentially perpetuate your well-being.

Practices like concentration meditation exemplify this pillar. Here, one directs attention to a single object (such as the breath), gently redirecting the mind when it wanders. This exercise helps stabilize attention and reduce distractibility.

#### 2. Open awareness

The second pillar focuses on broadening awareness to include a wider spectrum of experiences without becoming entangled in them.

When you consciously bring something into awareness, you *maintain* a specific neural firing pattern for an extended period.

Open awareness involves mindfulness meditation, in which one observes thoughts, emotions, and physical sensations nonjudgmentally. The practice of open awareness fosters mental spaciousness and adaptability. Mindfulness, or consciousness is crucial in facilitating change because it stabilizes newly-forged neural firing patterns, and allows for the integration of new information and experiences, potentially leading to lasting alterations in brain structure and function.

### 3. Kind intention

The third pillar emphasizes the importance of bringing a kind, compassionate attitude toward the internal world, toward others, and toward life in general. It is based on self-compassion or inner-compassion. The act of kind intention includes practices like loving-kindness meditation, where one directs well-wishes towards oneself and others. Kind intention helps to counter self-criticism and promote a sense of connection and empathy.

### Benefits of Three-pillar Practice

Integrating the three pillars into daily life can lead to what Siegel describes as an "integrated brain," characterized by enhanced cognitive, emotional, and social capabilities, more balanced emotional responses, improved stress resilience, better decision-making, and improved relationships. Integration supports individual health, happiness, well-being, and broader social harmony. Somatonous practice fosters a sense of gratitude, ease, and connectedness, contributing to overall mental health and a more integrated sense of self.

In addition to enhancing brain structure and function, these practices offer substantial physiological benefits by reducing cortisol levels, enhancing immune function, and improving cardiovascular risk factors. They also reduce inflammation by stimulating epigenetic changes in the chromosomes that repair and maintain the ends of chromosomes, called telomeres, slowing the aging process.

In addition, the practice helps balance the sympathetic and parasympathetic nervous systems, improving heart rate variability coherence. Heart rate variability reflects the balance between the sympathetic (fight-or-flight) and parasympathetic (rest-and-digest) nervous systems, with higher variability indicating better autonomic balance and adaptability to stress. Heart rate variability coherence refers to a state of synchronization between heart rhythm patterns, breathing, and other physiological systems. In this state, the heart rate varies in a smooth, rhythmic pattern, typically aligning with the breath. This coherence is associated with improved physical and mental well-being, including reduced stress, enhanced cognitive function, and better emotional regulation.

By engaging in the three-pillar practice, you can employ the resources of your own conscious mental activities to positively impact your physical well-being.

### Three-pillar Sauna Practice

Sauna practice is a unique and powerful form of somatonous practice and integration. The sauna's intense heat creates an ideal setting for linking different aspects of our experience—such as bodily sensations, emotions, thoughts, and memories—into a coherent whole. this practice. With heightened physical sensation, the mind is drawn to the present moment, making it easy to observe and connect various elements of consciousness. The sauna's heat induces focused awareness, similar to meditation, where different domains of experience can be accessed and integrated.

### *Heat-enhanced focused attention*

The sauna's enclosed, dimly lit space creates a mild sensory deprivation environment ideal for introspection. Naturally limiting external stimuli guides attention inward. You become more attuned to bodily sensations, thoughts, and emotions overlooked in daily life.

Concentrating on the sensations of heat is an opportunity to further focus attention. Focusing on physiological sensations like heat on the skin, the rhythm of breathing, or sweating helps anchor awareness. This inward focus can help integrate disconnected aspects of self, fostering a sense of wholeness and authenticity.

The intense heat of the sauna makes it an ideal environment to practice focusing solely on bodily sensations, helping to train the mind to remain present and not wander. This state of heightened attention aligns with Siegel's "guiding flow" concept and the principle that directed attention can promote neural growth and change. Regular practice in the sauna may improve attentional stability, potentially leading to lasting changes in focus and self-awareness even outside the sauna.

### Heat-enhanced open awareness

As the body acclimates to the sauna's heat, the parasympathetic nervous system is activated, promoting a state of "rest and digest." This response reduces heart rate, slows breathing, and decreases muscle tension. These physical changes correlate with calming mental activity, making transitioning into a state of open awareness easier. This physiological shift naturally supports a less reactive, more open state of awareness in which it is more natural to allow sensations, thoughts, and emotions to flow freely without attachment or judgment. The body's reduced stress response enables a non-reactive observation of experiences.

For instance, one might become aware of varying heat sensations across the body without feeling compelled to change or react to them. Similarly, thoughts about daily events or anticipations may arise and pass without triggering the usual chain of reactive thinking or emotion.

This parasympathetic-supported state of awareness in the sauna can help train the mind to maintain a non-reactive stance even when faced with potentially uncomfortable or challenging physical and mental experiences. Consistent practice in non-reactive awareness potentially carries over into daily life situations.

### Heat-enhanced kind intention

The state of non-reactive awareness induced in the sauna creates an ideal setting for cultivating kind intentions. As you learn to observe experience without immediate reaction to the heat and physical discomfort, you develop a capacity for acceptance and self-compassion. This non-reactive stance allows a more forgiving and gentle response to challenging sensations, thoughts, and emotions. From this place of acceptance, you can more easily direct thoughts of kindness towards yourself, appreciating your body's resilience in the face of discomfort. This self-directed kindness forms the foundation for extending compassion to others.

The shared experience of the sauna with others, stripped of social pretenses, highlights our common humanity and vulnerability. Non-reactive awareness in our interactions with others allows us to observe this shared experience without defensiveness, naturally fostering empathy and connection. Coupling non-reactive awareness with kind intention enhances our capacity for empathy and compassion, potentially carrying over into daily life.

### Heat-enhanced Integration

The psychological concept of integration emphasizes the interconnectedness of mind and body, viewing symptoms not as isolated issues but as manifestations of systemic dysregulation. This holistic perspective aligns closely with emerging research on the mind-body connection and the complex interplay between psychological states and physical health.

As my case revealed, what initially presented as discrete symptoms affecting specific body systems—insomnia, tachycardia, and mood disturbances—were in reality expressions of dysregulation across my body's multiple systems. Rather than treating each symptom in isolation, an integrative, somatonous approach suggests that these symptoms stem from common underlying factors, such as chronic stress, inflammation, or autonomic nervous system imbalance.

By inducing a controlled stress response, sauna use impacts multiple bodily systems simultaneously—promoting cardiovascular health, enhancing detoxification pathways, modulating the immune system, and potentially improving mood and cognitive function. This multifaceted intervention addresses the body as an integrated whole, potentially rebalancing systems that have fallen out of homeostasis.

By viewing health through this lens of integration, we can better understand how seemingly disparate symptoms may be interconnected and how holistic interventions like sauna use can have wide-ranging benefits across both physical and mental domains.

### Sauna savasana

Savasana, commonly known as Corpse Pose, is the final resting posture in a yoga practice where one lies still on the back, allowing the body and mind to fully relax and stabilize itself in a heightened state of integration and harmony. I take a short savasana of several minutes after cooling off from each interval. When I re-enter the sauna, I lie in a state of bodily relaxation and mental integration, which allows me to internalize a stable sense of calm.

**Conclusion**

The rhythmic alternation between heat and cool, activity and rest, solitude and sociality in the sauna mirrors the natural oscillations of conditions of the environment and our adaptive responses to them. This intentional exposure to contrasting states supports integration, fostering balance and resilience in facing life's challenges. By engaging in this practice, you can develop a more adaptive and flexible response to stress, enhancing your overall well-being and capacity to navigate life's ups and downs.

Ultimately, the spiritual essence of sauna practice lies in its power to integrate body, mind, and spirit within a context of warmth, stillness, and connection. The sauna transcends its physical structure to become a sacred space for expanding consciousness and deepening our sense of universal belonging. This integration process unites us with ourselves, each other, and the broader web of life, fostering a profound sense of interconnectedness. In this way, the sauna experience serves as a microcosm of broader spiritual practices, offering a tangible path to wholeness and unity that can extend far beyond the confines of the sauna itself.

# 21. SAUNA SOCIALITY
## FINDING A SAUNA KULA

"I define connection as the energy that exists between people when they feel seen, heard, and valued; when they can give and receive without judgment; and when they derive sustenance and strength from the relationship."

— Brené Brown

K*ula* is the Sanskrit word for community. It refers to a group of people united by a common practice or spiritual path. The ancient concept of kula finds new relevance in the shared rituals and routines of sauna practice.

The profound relaxation and mental clarity induced by the sauna experience create an ideal environment for forming and strengthening social connections. As individuals enter a meditative, trance-like state, the intense heat and shared vulnerability break down social barriers, fostering trust and openness among participants. This relaxed state often leads to more authentic, meaningful conversations.

The sense of physical and mental renewal experienced in the sauna becomes a shared journey, creating a bond among those who go through it together. This vulnerability and openness can lead to deeper connections, understanding, and empathy among sauna participants. The environment of quiet contemplation allows for comfortable silences, deepening connections on an intuitive level.

### Inclusivity

The sauna is a great equalizer, where people from all walks of life come together on the same terms, stripped of their social roles and status. In this intimate and egalitarian setting, barriers dissolve, and genuine human connection can flourish. The relaxed, intimate setting encourages conversation and sharing of personal stories and experiences. As individuals sit together in the heat, they often find themselves opening up to one another in ways they might not in other social settings. Social bonds form between people of different ages, cultures, and backgrounds. Connections to others that transcend age, background, and culture enrich our lives by broadening our perspectives and fostering empathy.

### Community

Regular sauna sessions can evolve into a shared ritual, fostering a sense of community and belonging. As you establish a sauna routine, you will encounter others who participate regularly.

Over time, through repeated encounters, strangers become acquaintances, and acquaintances become friends. This familiarity breeds a sense of camaraderie and connection as participants learn one another's stories and come to recognize and appreciate their presence.

Over time, this shared routine can lead to a tight-knit community where individuals look forward to seeing each other and sharing the sauna experience. This organic space for the growth of relationships and the strengthening of community has always been a vital aspect of the sauna experience. It is one of the profound benefits of the practice.

### Unity

The shared physical experience of the sauna is conducive to creating a sense of unity and togetherness. As participants endure the heat together, they develop a sense of collective accomplishment and resilience. This shared challenge can foster a sense of solidarity and support among sauna-goers as they encourage and motivate one another to push through the discomfort in the cause of self-renewal. The feeling of interconnectedness with others strengthens and empowers us.

**The Basic Human Need for Connection**

The importance of these social connections formed in the sauna goes beyond mere companionship. From an evolutionary standpoint, they serve a crucial function in maintaining our cognitive and social capacities. Our ability to form and strengthen social bonds has been a critical factor in human evolution, shaping the development of our brains, particularly the prefrontal cortex. This region, responsible for complex social cognition, thrives on regular social interaction. Just as the heat of the sauna maintains our physical capacities, its social environment stimulates our social-cognitive abilities, which are vital for our overall well-being.

Moreover, the sauna environment provides an ideal setting for social bonding that anthropologists call "vocal grooming." This concept, proposed by British anthropologist Robin Dunbar, offers insights into how language may have evolved as a more efficient means of maintaining social bonds in larger groups, replacing the physical grooming behavior observed in lower primates (Dunbar, 1996). Dunbar's theory posits that as early hominids evolved and their group sizes increased, the time required for physical grooming to maintain group cohesion became increasingly challenging. Early hominids began using vocalizations to overcome the constraints of the larger social group, which eventually evolved into language as a more efficient way to interact with multiple group members simultaneously, share information, and express emotions, all of which contribute to social bonding.

The relaxed, intimate setting of the sauna encourages open communication and sharing, mirroring the conditions our ancestors might have experienced during rest periods after hunts or around evening fires, where we can participate in vocal grooming. This modern manifestation of community in the sauna setting has deep roots in our evolutionary past, reflecting fundamental aspects of human social development.

**An Antidote to Isolation**

The communal aspect of the sauna experience is particularly relevant in today's society, where loneliness and social isolation have become widespread concerns. In an age where technology has made it easier to connect virtually, many people feel disconnected from genuine human interaction. The U.S. Surgeon General has recently announced this issue as a public health crisis, highlighting the profound impact of disconnection on both mental and physical well-being. The sauna is a conducive environment for social connections rarely encountered in modern life.

## My Sauna Kula

I embarked on my sauna journey during a period of profound personal challenge. Emerging from years of social isolation and the aftermath of a profoundly unhealthy marriage, I found myself at a dark crossroads. My mental well-being was fragile, and I was adrift in a new world in which I felt isolated and afraid.

In this context, my sauna routine unexpectedly became a space for reconnection with others and, ultimately, with myself. At first, during my solitary visits, I encountered strangers in the darkness of an unfamiliar and uncomfortable space. But as my routine became established and I learned to welcome the heat, these strangers became familiar acquaintances.

In the safe, intimate space of the sauna, I felt the courage to share my story. These women listened compassionately and without judgment, offering empathy and understanding that nourished my hungry soul.

As we shared our stories of struggle, we uncovered common threads of experience and resilience and found mutual support and strength. Our conversations spanned beyond the challenges of our past stories to encompass present challenges and hopeful aspirations. Over time, these encounters blossomed into friendships with women I now affectionately call my *sauna sisters*.

This unexpected community came at the darkest hours of my life when I most needed it. My sauna sisters became a lifeline I could hold onto as I pulled myself forward in the journey of healing and spiritual rebirth.

## Expand Your Social World

As you develop a consistent sauna practice, you'll become part of an evolving social ecosystem. As your sauna routine becomes a fixture in your life, you will find a kula, and it will play a role in satisfying your enduring need for community, ritual, and shared experience. Your kula will become a source of strength, support, and social connection that enriches your life.

# PART FIVE

## THE END. YOUR BEGINNING.

As we near the conclusion of our exploration of the world of the sauna, we find ourselves not at an end but at the threshold of a new beginning. The knowledge and insights you've gained are fuel for your future journey. As you read these final chapters, remember that while this book may end, your sauna personal sauna narrative is just beginning.

Envision these final chapters as a bridge between the comprehensive foundation we've built together and the limitless potential of your future sauna experiences. Your journey into the transformative sauna world could become a lifelong adventure, rich with opportunities for health, growth, and self-discovery. Embrace this new beginning with curiosity, openness, and enthusiasm, and know that profound experiences lie in the sauna practice ahead of you.

# 22. MY SAUNA STORY: A CONCLUSION

My sauna practice has considerably enriched my life over the past three years.

I've successfully reversed many symptoms I once suffered as a result of nervous system dysfunction, including symptoms of PTSD, migraines, insomnia, anxiety, and depression.

I've also improved my cardiovascular fitness, as evidenced by a 30-point reduction in my heart rate and my ability to maintain aerobic endurance for 60 minutes a day at vigorous intensity, which, notably, I developed after the age of 60. My vigorous daily cardiovascular workout allows my heart to beat 40 times more than at rest, which means that 56 additional gallons of blood are circulating through my system, saturating my cells with oxygen.

My immunity has also improved. I've effectively avoided illness of any kind for over three years. At the first sign of symptoms, an extended sauna session has consistently thwarted the onset of illness.

Over three years of sauna practice, I've experienced profound improvements in my overall mental well-being. The practice has become essential for stress management, offering daily calm and introspection. This improved mental clarity and resilience have positively impacted my decision-making, relationships, and life satisfaction. The ripple effects of better mental health are extensive, influencing career performance and personal life in ways that defy simple economic valuation. While it's difficult to assign a monetary value to peace of mind and emotional stability, these benefits undoubtedly contribute to a richer, more fulfilling life experience, complementing the economic advantages of sauna therapy.

While the sauna offers numerous benefits, it's important to understand that it's not a magic solution for complex health issues. Significant bodily dysfunctions often result from the body's maladaptive responses to environmental stressors over time, and healing is gradual. In my case, although most symptoms have subsided, the effects of chronic stress continue to linger. My cortisol levels start at the higher end of average in the morning, but instead of following a healthy decline throughout the day, they spike to more than three times higher than average in the afternoon. A nighttime sauna session reduces cortisol dramatically, yet levels remain nearly three times higher than normal at night. Despite these challenges, I remain cautiously optimistic that my nervous system will gradually recalibrate with consistent sauna practice and patience, restoring natural balance. This journey toward healing underscores the importance of persistence and realistic expectations in addressing long-standing health issues.

Reflecting on my sauna practice, have profound gratitude for its potential to safeguard my future health and financial well-being. By consistently using the sauna, I'm not just enjoying immediate benefits; I'm making a long-term investment in disease prevention and longevity. The prospect of maintaining better health as I age means I will be more likely to enjoy an active, independent retirement without the burden of disease and associated healthcare costs. The thought of avoiding the devastating costs associated with common chronic diseases is both comforting and empowering. Heart disease, diabetes, and cancer can drain savings and derail retirement plans, not to mention cause immeasurable suffering. My daily sauna sessions could save hundreds of thousands of dollars in future medical expenses by reducing my risk for these conditions.

My sauna lifestyle approach has translated into tangible economic benefits as well. I've significantly changed my home energy use by incorporating regular sauna sessions at my local gym into my routine. Because I shower at the gym, I keep my water heater off during the summer and at a lower temperature in winter. This adjustment saves 14-18% on home energy costs typically associated with water heating. My increased heat tolerance allows me to forgo air conditioning entirely in the summer, even during the hottest days, saving an additional 20% on household energy bills in summer. Given my body's improved thermo-regulatory capacities and my new appreciation of the health benefits of cold exposure, I can keep the temperature in my home between 68-70° in winter, lowering heating expenses.

This sustainable approach aligns perfectly with my financial stability and personal freedom goals. While it's impossible to predict the exact impact, I'm confident that my committed sauna practice sets me up for a healthier, more economically secure future. The peace of mind this brings—knowing I'm actively working to avoid the physical and finan-cial toll of chronic disease—is truly invaluable.

Compared to these substantial health improvements and cost savings, the expense of my sauna practice—approximately 2¢ per minute based on a $60 monthly gym membership—is minimal. My sauna prac-tice has demonstrated significant potential for promoting a more economically sustainable and minimalist lifestyle. It shows how sauna practice can offer improved health and financial sustainability, providing a compelling model for individuals seeking to optimize their well-being and budget.

While my experience is individual, it suggests that sauna therapy could have a dramatic positive economic impact when adopted more widely. It could provide a valuable tool for individuals and families seeking to live sustainably without compromising personal wellness.

In conclusion, my journey with sauna therapy is a compelling case study, illustrating its potential for personal transformation and fostering a more economically sustainable and minimalist lifestyle.

# CONGRATULATIONS!

You've completed this exploration of heat therapy and its potential benefits for your physical, mental, and spiritual well-being. As you begin to incorporate these practices into your life, consider sharing your experiences to help others on their own wellness journeys.

**Share Your Insights**

Your feedback can be invaluable to others seeking to:

• Enhance their physical health
• Cultivate mental clarity
• Explore spiritual growth
• Promote overall longevity

**Leave a Review**

If you found value in this book, please consider leaving a review. Your insights can guide fellow readers toward potentially life-changing practices.

To share your review, simply scan the QR code below or visit https://rb.gy/p18asb.

Thank you for your time, openness, and willingness to share your experience with others. May your journey continue to be one of growth and discovery.

Warmest regards,

Dr. Cynthia McCallister

# 23. CONCLUSION
## EMBRACING THE SAUNA WAY OF LIFE

As we conclude our exploration into the transformative power of sauna and heat therapy, we come to a pivotal juncture in our understanding of human wellness. Throughout this book, we have revealed the profound potential of harnessing intense heat as a catalyst for adaptation and resilience. Our central thesis has been bold yet simple: regular, sustained exposure to the extreme temperatures of the sauna can unlock a cascade of benefits that extend far beyond physical comfort.

In this concluding chapter, we will synthesize the insights gained throughout the journey to frame a new paradigm for understanding and harnessing the power of heat as a revolution in wellness, one that recognizes the sauna not just as a luxury but as a fundamental tool for health, longevity, and personal transformation. The sauna tradition, ancient as it is, still has new lessons to teach us about our bodies, our health, and our capacity for adaptation.

### Harnessing the Therapeutic Effects of Heat

In this book, we've delved deep into the science and practice of sauna use, revealing how intense heat is a powerful tool for physical health by stimulating activity across all body systems. The sauna's heat is a hormetic stressor, challenging our bodies to adapt, grow stronger, and become more resilient.

The approach presented in this book, centered around the protocol I developed for sauna-based cardiovascular training (S-CET), harnesses the power of heat for healing. By subjecting the body to prolonged durations of high levels of heat stress in the dry sauna that are carefully managed in intervals with cold exposure techniques, this method aims to extend the body's tolerance, improve resilience, and trigger profound physiological adaptations at the cellular level that positively impact all of the body's systems.

## Reconsidering Conventional Understandings of Health and Disease

The innovative approach to heat as a source of therapy invites us to reconsider our modern understanding of health and disease. We often view the progression of lifestyle-related illnesses as an inevitable destiny. Conditions such as cardiovascular disease, dementia (including Alzheimer's), mental illness, cancer, and diabetes are typically managed in stages of increasing medical intervention to delay the most severe manifestations of disease until the later stages of life.

This book challenges this conventional perspective, offering a paradigm shift in how we approach these diseases of modern living. Rather than accepting disease as an inevitable destiny, this work encourages us to view it as a state of bodily dysregulation—one in which symptoms and root causes can be addressed and potentially reversed through controlled exposure to heat stress combined with complementary lifestyle practices.

This disruptive approach holds promise as a preventative measure against lifestyle diseases and a potential intervention to reverse existing disease processes, offering a new frontier in our quest for holistic health and longevity.

## Mental Well-being and Spiritual Rebirth

As we've discovered, the impact of intense heat reaches far more profound than physical wellness alone. It touches the very core of our mental and emotional well-being, offering a path to rejuvenation that encompasses body, mind, and spirit.

As you embark upon your sauna journey, I'm sure you will find that the most profound reward is heat as a source of mental rejuvenation. The sauna environment provokes a heat-induced altered consciousness and offers isolation from daily distractions, creating an environment conducive to transcendent experiences. Stress seems to dissolve, mental clarity sharpens, and emotional equilibrium is restored. These moments of heightened awareness and introspection offer opportunities for deep personal reflection. I'm sure you'll find that these combined effects will contribute significantly to overall mental well-being, transforming the sauna from a basic physical health practice into a powerful tool for psychological growth and emotional balance. The sauna's heat, it turns out, not only warms the body but also soothes and invigorates the mind, offering a holistic approach to wellness that addresses both physical and mental health.

**Longevity**

Tying these threads together is the optimistic prospect of expansive longevity. By regularly subjecting ourselves to intense heat, we activate cellular processes that stimulate longevity pathways in our bodies. This heat-induced cellular response may hold the key to not only extending our lifespan but also enhancing the quality of our years. The controlled stress of heat exposure triggers adaptive mechanisms at the molecular level, potentially fortifying our cells against age-related decline and promoting overall resilience. This approach offers a promising avenue for harnessing our body's innate ability to repair and rejuvenate, potentially unlocking a longer, healthier life. As we embrace heat as a tool for wellness, we open the door to a future where longevity is not just about adding years to life but adding life to years.

**Renewing Our Primordial Relationship With Heat**

Throughout this journey, we've uncovered an intriguing contrast between the standard cultural narrative surrounding heat and the emerging research on controlled heat exposure. Media and public health messaging often focus on the dangers of extreme temperatures, with frequent warnings about heat waves and the importance of avoiding overexposure. These cautionary messages serve a vital purpose in protecting public health, especially during extreme weather events. However, our exploration has revealed that this perspective tells only part of the story.

The other part, which we've examined in depth, suggests that intentional, controlled heat exposure, such as that experienced in a sauna, may offer significant health benefits. From potential improvements in cardiovascular health and longevity to enhanced mental clarity and emotional balance, the controlled use of heat presents a more nuanced picture than the prevailing narrative might suggest. Without dismissing the real dangers of excessive heat exposure, we propose a more balanced understanding. By considering both the risks and potential benefits, we can develop a more comprehensive approach to heat that respects its power while also harnessing its possible advantages for human health and well-being.

On this threshold of a new understanding, it becomes clear that we need to reframe our relationship with heat. Heat shouldn't be solely viewed as a threat to be avoided but rather as a powerful ally in the quest for optimal wellness. By approaching heat exposure with the same intentionality and respect we afford to rest, exercise, and nutrition, we unlock a potent tool for enhancing both physical and mental well-being. It's time to shed our misplaced fear of heat and embrace it as a valuable component of a holistic approach to health, tapping into an often-overlooked dimension of human adaptability that has supported our species for millennia.

**Empowerment**

This exploration has equipped you with the knowledge and tools to establish your transformative sauna practice. This practice is a lifelong gift of proactive well-being. Once you develop your body's capacity to tolerate extended heat exposure, you acquire a versatile tool that empowers you to take control of your physical and mental health, which you can use for a lifetime. By embracing regular sauna use, you're not just adopting a wellness routine but investing in a sustainable, self-directed approach to health and well-being.

As you reflect on the insights gained from this book, remember that the power to harness intense heat for transformative purposes is in your hands. Whether you're stepping into a sauna for the first time or deepening an established practice, approach each session with intention and awareness. Listen to your body, push your limits gradually, and stay open to the physical, mental, and spiritual changes that unfold before you. There's joy to be had in the journey.

**Advocacy**

As you experience the benefits of sauna therapy firsthand, I urge you to become an advocate for this ancient practice. Heat can heal. So, share your knowledge and experiences with friends and family. By spreading the sauna gospel, you can help others discover the path to improved health and well-being and help make sauna practice mainstream.

**Conclusion**

As we look to the future, it's clear that sauna practice aligns with a growing desire for natural, holistic health and personal development approaches. As a tool for comprehensive transformation, the sauna offers potential benefits that span the physical, mental, and spiritual realms. I am grateful you have chosen to join the movement for self-empowered wellness.

In closing, thank you for the privilege of sharing my sauna journey. I hope this book inspires you to harness the transformative power of intense heat and guides you toward enhanced physical health, mental well-being, spiritual rebirth, and the promise of expansive longevity.

———

*Namaste*

# Appendix A
## Sauna Culture Connections and Resources

The following appendices provide a curated list of online resources In today's digital age, sauna traditions and modern practices are widely discussed, shared, and celebrated across various social media platforms and dedicated websites. This appendix provides a curated list of online resources for anyone interested in sauna culture. It offers a wealth of information for those looking to deepen their understanding of sauna culture, connect with fellow enthusiasts, or find inspiration for their sauna experiences.

The appendices are organized by platform type, including popular social media sites like Instagram and Facebook, video-sharing platforms like YouTube, informative websites, and discussion forums like Reddit.

**Instagram:**
@saunatimes
@saunareviews
@finnishsaunalife
@saunafreaks
@sauna_nomad
@worldsaunaforum
@sweatandsteam
@saunaexperience

**YouTube:**
Sauna Times channel
Finnmark Sauna
Sauna From Finland channel
Saunatalk with Glenn
Sauna Lifestyle
The Sauna Show
**Facebook Groups:**
Sauna Enthusiasts
Mobile Sauna Community
International Sauna Association
Sauna Builders and DIY
Outdoor Sauna Enthusiasts
**Podcasts and Audio Content**
"Sauna Talk" podcast
"Heat It Up: The Sauna Podcast"
"Sweat It Out: Sauna Health and Wellness"
"Finnish Sauna Stories"
**Mobile Applications:**
Sauna Timer Pro
SaunaMaster
Sauna Tracker
Virtual Sauna Experience
Sauna Temp Monitor
**Websites:**
finnishsauna.fi
nordicsaunas.com
saunatimes.com
saunascape.com
saunasite.com
thesaunalife.com
saunahealth.org
saunasessions.com
saunadigest.com
**Reddit:**
- r/Sauna

**Twitter:**

@SaunaTimes

@SaunaSessions

@SaunaScience

@SaunaWisdom

@GlobalSaunaClub

**Pinterest:**

Sauna Design boards

Sauna Health Benefits boards

DIY Sauna Construction boards

Sauna Interior Design Ideas

**Academic and Research Resources**

PubMed Central (search for sauna-related studies)

ResearchGate (sauna research papers)

JSTOR (articles on sauna culture and history)

ScienceDirect (scientific studies on sauna benefits)

**Online Sauna Retailers:**

saunastore.com

finnleo.com

almostheaven.com

**Sauna Associations Websites:**

International Sauna Association (www.saunainternational.org)

North American Sauna Society (www.northamericansaunasociety.com)

**Sauna Event Calendars:**

World Sauna Forum events

Local sauna meetups and gatherings

**Sauna Design and Architecture:**

Houzz.com (sauna design ideas)

Architizer.com (innovative sauna architecture)

# APPENDIX B
## STARTING A SAUNA CO-OP

A sauna co-op is a community-driven initiative where individuals collectively own, operate, and maintain a sauna facility. This cooperative model allows members to share the costs, responsibilities, and benefits of having a high-quality sauna without the full financial burden of individual ownership. Members typically contribute to initial setup costs, ongoing maintenance, and operational expenses while enjoying scheduled facility access. Sauna co-ops are often governed democratically, with members making decisions about operations and improvements. They can range from small groups sharing a single sauna to larger organizations with multiple facilities. Beyond the practical benefits, sauna co-ops foster a sense of community among members who share an interest in sauna culture. This approach offers a middle ground between public saunas and private home installations, providing an affordable, community-oriented solution for regular sauna use. This unique idea that combines the social and health benefits of sauna use with a cooperative business model.

Here's a step-by-step guide to get you started:

1. Research and Planning

Market Research: Understand the demand for a sauna in your area.

Look into potential competitors and assess what they offer. Determine your target market (e.g., health enthusiasts, families, older adults).

Business Model: Decide how the co-op will operate. Most co-ops are owned and run by members who contribute to the capital and decision-making processes. Determine if the sauna will be member-only or open to the public for additional revenue.

Legal Structure: Research the legal requirements for starting a co-op in your region. This typically includes registering the business, obtaining necessary licenses, and understanding health and safety regulations specific to saunas.

2. Membership and Community Engagement

Recruit Initial Members: You'll need a core group of founding members. These individuals can help with startup tasks and contribute to the initial capital needed.

Community Outreach: Engage with the local community through events, social media, and local advertising. Highlight the benefits of joining the co-op, such as ownership rights, health benefits, and a sense of community.

Membership Structure: Define the membership fees, benefits, and responsibilities. Consider offering different levels of membership based on usage, such as unlimited monthly access or pay-per-visit rates.

3. Location and Setup

Location: Find a suitable location for the sauna. Consider factors like accessibility, size, and local zoning laws.

Facility Requirements: Depending on your budget and preferences, you may build a new facility or adapt an existing one. Include space for changing rooms, showers, and a relaxation area.

Equipment: Purchase or lease sauna equipment. Ensure that it meets safety standards and is efficient to operate.

4. Financing

Startup Capital: Funding can come from member contributions, small business loans, or grants. Detailed financial planning is crucial.

Budget Management: Prepare a detailed budget that includes construction or renovation costs, operational expenses, and marketing.

5. Operations and Management

Hiring Staff: Depending on the size of your co-op, you may need to hire staff for daily operations, maintenance, and customer service.

Software and Tools: Implement management software for bookings, memberships, and financial tracking.

Policies and Procedures: Develop clear policies for usage, membership, and health and safety compliance.

6. Marketing and Growth

Launch Marketing: Organize a grand opening event to attract initial members and press coverage. Offer introductory discounts or bundle packages.

Ongoing Promotion: Maintain visibility with regular marketing efforts, partnerships with local businesses, and special events.

Feedback and Adaptation: Keep in touch with members for feedback to continuously improve the services and address any issues.

7. Sustaining the Co-op

Regular Member Meetings: As a co-op, regular meetings to discuss the management, financial status, and strategic direction are essential.

Transparency and Inclusion: Ensure all members feel included in the decision-making process and have access to financial and operational updates.

By following these steps, you can establish a successful sauna co-op that benefits both its members and the broader community.

# Appendix C
## Organizing a Community Sauna Wellness Initiative

Bringing a sauna to your community can be a transformative wellness initiative promoting physical and mental health. This appendix outlines essential steps for organizing such a project. By following these guidelines, community members can collaborate to create a valuable wellness resource enhancing overall quality of life.

1. Define Benefits and Goals

Gather credible information on sauna health benefits, including scientific studies. Clearly define your goal: one public sauna, multiple saunas, or integration into existing facilities?

2. Engage Health Experts and Stakeholders

Consult health professionals, wellness experts, and local health departments for support and endorsements. Their opinions lend credibility.

3. Build a Core Team

Assemble passionate individuals who believe in community sauna benefits. This team will help plan, engage, and execute strategies.

4. Community Engagement and Feedback

Host informational sessions to introduce sauna benefits. Gather feedback, gauge interest, and encourage community input on integrating saunas.

5. Develop a Proposal

Create a detailed proposal based on research, health professional endorsements, and community feedback. Include locations, costs, funding sources, timeline, and address concerns.

6. Identify Funding Opportunities

Explore options like local government budgets, health grants, crowdfunding, or partnerships. Include cost analysis and potential funding sources in the proposal.

7. Lobby Local Government

Present your proposal to officials and bodies. Prepare to answer questions about benefits and logistics.

8. Use Media and Social Campaigns

Generate public support through local media and social platforms. Share stories, updates, and calls to action.

9. Organize Demonstrations or Trials

If possible, organize a temporary sauna event to demonstrate benfits and sway opinion.

10. Monitor and Adapt

Keep the community informed and adapt strategies based on feedback and developments.

11. Celebrate and Expand

Once successful, celebrate with supporters and consider advocating for more wellness facilities.

# References

American Heart Association. (n.d.). Heart attack and stroke symptoms. Heart.org. https://www.heart.org/

American Heart Association. (2017). Cardiovascular disease: A costly burden for America — Projections through 2035. https://www.heart.org/-/media/files/about-us/policy-research/fact-sheets/ucm_491543.pdf

Ben-Dor, M., Sirtoli, R., & Barkai, R. (2021). The evolution of the human trophic level during the Pleistocene. American Journal of Physical Anthropology. https://doi.org/10.1002/ajpa.24247

Bramble, D. M. & Lieberman, D. E. (2004). Endurance running and the evolution of *Homo*. Nature 432, 345–352.

Chen, X., Barywani, S. B., Hansson, P. O., Thunström, E., Rosengren, A., & Fu, M. (2017). Resting heart rate in cardiovascular disease. Journal of the American College of Cardiology, 70(9), 1176-1186. https://doi.org/10.1016/j.jacc.2017.07.720

Chevalier, C., Kieser, S., Çolakoğlu, M., Hadadi, N., Brun, J., Rigo, D., Suárez-Zamorano, N., Spiljar, M., Fabbiano, S., Busse, B., Ivanišević, J., Macpherson, A., Bonnet, N., & Trajkovski, M. (2020). Warmth prevents bone loss through the gut microbiota. Cell Metabolism. https://doi.org/10.1016/j.cmet.2020.08.012

Dunbar, R. (1996). Grooming, gossip and the evolution of language. Harvard University Press.

Dunbar, R. I. M. (1992). Neocortex size as a constraint on group size in primates. Journal of Human Evolution, 22(6), 469-493.

The Global BMI Mortality Collaboration. (2016). Body-mass index and all-cause mortality: Individual-participant-data meta-analysis of 239 prospective studies in four continents. The Lancet, 388(10046), 776-786. https://doi.org/10.1016/S0140-6736(16)30175-1

Gurven, M., & Kaplan, H. (2007). Longevity among hunter-gatherers: A cross-cultural examination. Population and Development Review, 33(2), 321–365.

Henderson, K. N., Killen, L. G., O'Neal, E. K., & Waldman, H. S. (2021). The cardiometabolic health benefits of sauna exposure in individuals with high-stress occupations. A mechanistic review. International Journal of Environmental Research and Public Health, 18(3), 1105. https://doi.org/10.3390/ijerph18031105

Jensen, M. T., Suadicani, P., Hein, H. O., & Gyntelberg, F. (2013). Elevated resting heart rate, physical fitness and all-cause mortality: A 16-year follow-up in the Copenhagen Male Study. Heart, 99(12), 882-887.

Kaplan, H., Gangestad, S., Gurven, M., Lancaster, J., Mueller, T., & Robson, A. (2007). The evolution of diet, brain and life history among primates and humans. In W. Roebroeks (Ed.), Guts and brains: An integrative approach to the hominin record (pp. 47–48). Leiden University Press.

Kaplan, H., Hill, K., Lancaster, J., & Hurtado, A. M. (2000). A theory of human life history evolution: Diet, intelligence, and longevity. Evolutionary Anthropology Issues News and Reviews, 9(4), 156–185.

Kiani, A. K., Dhuli, K., Donato, K., Aquilanti, B., Velluti, V., Matera, G., Iaconelli, A., Connelly, S. T., Bellinato, F., Gisondi, P., & Bertelli, M. (2022). Main nutritional deficiencies. Journal of Preventive Medicine and Hygiene, 63(2 Suppl 3), E93–E101. https://doi.org/10.15167/2421-4248/jpmh2022.63.2S3.2752

Kunutsor, S. K., Jae, S. Y., & Laukkanen, J. A. (2022). Frequent sauna bathing offsets the increased risk of death due to low socioeconomic status: A prospective cohort study of middle-aged and older men. Experimental Gerontology, 167, 111906. https://doi.org/10.1016/j.exger.2022.111906

Kunutsor, S. K., Laukkanen, T., & Laukkanen, J. A. (2018). Longitudinal associations of sauna bathing with inflammation and oxidative stress: The KIHD prospective cohort study. Annals of Medicine, 50(5), 437-442.

Lake, I. (2021). Nutritional ketosis is well-tolerated, even in type 1 diabetes: The Zero-Five100 Project; A proof-of-concept study. Current Opinion in Endocrinology & Diabetes and Obesity, 28(5), 453-462. https://doi.org/10.1097/MED.0000000000000666

Laukkanen, T., Khan, H., Zaccardi, F., & Laukkanen, J. A. (2015). Association between sauna bathing and fatal cardiovascular and all-cause mortality events. JAMA Internal Medicine, 175(4), 542-548.

Laukkanen, T., Kunutsor, S., Kauhanen, J., & Laukkanen, J. A. (2018). Sauna bathing is associated with reduced cardiovascular mortality and improves risk prediction in men and women: A prospective cohort study. BMC Medicine, 16(1), 219.

Laukkanen, T., Laukkanen, J. A., & Kunutsor, S. K. (2018). Sauna bathing and risk of psychotic disorders: A prospective cohort study. Medical Principles and Practice, 27(6), 562–569. https://doi.org/10.1159/000493392

Mace, T. A., Zhong, L., Kilpatrick, C., Zynda, E., Lee, C. T., Capitano, M., Minderman, H., & Repasky, E. A. (2011). Differentiation of CD8+ T cells into effector cells is enhanced by physiological range hyperthermia. Journal of Leukocyte Biology, 90(5), 951–962. https://doi.org/10.1189/jlb.0511229

McCallister, C. (2022). A pedagogical design for human flourishing: Transforming schools with the McCallister Model. Routledge.

McCallister, C. (2011). Unison reading: Socially inclusive group instruction for equity and achievement. Corwin Press.

Passey, B. H., Levin, N. E., Cerling, T. E., Brown, F. H., & Eiler, J. M. (2010). High-temperature environments of human evolution in East Africa based on bond ordering in paleosol carbonates. Proceedings of the National Academy of Sciences, 107(25), 11245-11249. https://doi.org/10.1073/pnas.1001824107

Sadhguru. (n.d.). Nobody can do meditation! Inner Engineering. https://isha.sadhguru.org/en/sadhguru/mission/nobody-can-do-meditation

Seviiri, M., Milne, R. L., Giles, G. G., Hodge, A. M., English, D. R., Baglietto, L., ... & Dite, G. S. (2023). Resting heart rate, changes in resting heart rate, and overall and cause-specific mortality: A prospective cohort study. Heart, 109(7), 498-505.

Siegel, D. J. (2018). Aware: The science and practice of presence. TarcherPerigee.

Siegel, D. J. (2020). The power of awareness: Insights to create the life you want. Sounds True.

Siegel, D. J. (2012a). The developing mind: How relationships and the brain interact to shape who we are (2nd ed.). Guilford Press.

Siegel, D. J. (2012b). Pocket guide to interpersonal neurobiology: An integrative handbook of the mind. W.W. Norton & Company.

Sinclair, D. A., & LaPlante, M. D. (2019). Lifespan: Why we age—and why we don't have to. Atria Books.

Zaccardi, F., Laukkanen, T., Willeit, P., Kunutsor, S. K., Kauhanen, J., & Laukkanen, J. A. (2017). Sauna bathing and incident hypertension: A prospective cohort study. American Journal of Hypertension, 30(11), 1120-1125.